CU01335771

WALL PILATES FOR SENIORS

AN ILLUSTRATED GUIDE TO ENHANCE FLEXIBILITY,
LOSE WEIGHT, AND INCREASE BALANCE IN 21 DAYS!

RACHEL HADUCH

VITALITY SOLUTIONS PUBLISHING

Photography by
LESLIE HADUCH

This book is a guide to providing a simple yet detailed introduction to Wall Pilates for Seniors who want to live pain free, lose weight, improve posture, and feel better in their day-to-day life. There are clear and concise instructions for each exercise and its benefits, beginning with easy exercises and working through the book to more challenging postures. This book is a daily guide for people who want to improve their lives with an emphasis on creating a routine for improved exercise habits. Be inspired to dream big with many real-life stories from Elder Athletes who inspire the benefits of an active life.

CONTENTS

AUTHORS SECTION

Rachel Haduch and Leslie Haduch

This mother-and-daughter duo has always had a passion for healthy living and fitness. Leslie is a 72-year-young wellness-obsessed mother. She has found many ways to care for her body, bringing vitality into her life. Utilizing fitness and nutrition, she has cultivated impressive endurance and stamina in her workouts through dedication to herself in her golden years.

Leslie has proven that people can feel better in their bodies as they age through dedication to their goals. She has a morning workout practice that she adheres to, swims in the pool three times a week, and has healthy eating habits such as intermittent fasting that help the body stay in optimal shape.

As a home health aide, Rachel has cared for seniors on their health journey. She is writing this book because she realizes the need for caretaking the vitality of seniors' wellness so they can continue to be independent and strong.

These women are passionate about sharing the beneficial exercises of Wall Pilates. Rachel's experience with caring for Seniors and Leslie's lifetime of studying fitness and nutrition create a bridge of support for other Seniors to discover their inner strength and independence.

They aim to inspire confidence in those who feel helpless in their aging body, whose goal is to strengthen the mind-body connection with gentle Wall Pilates!

———

Enjoy this bonus exercise chart below to make this Wall Pilates Book easy to use and simple to incorporate into your everyday routine!

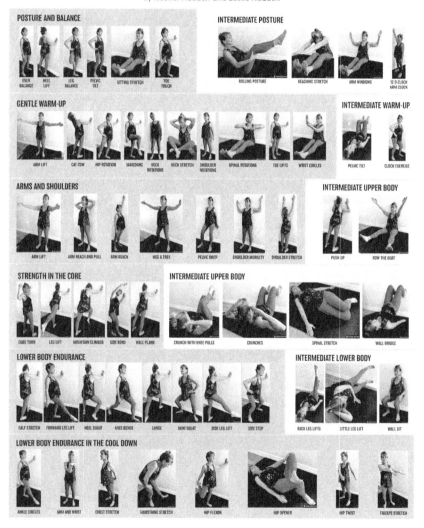

WALL PILATES FOR SENIORS
An Illustrated Guide to Enhance Flexibility, Lose Weight, and Increase Balance in 21 Days!
by Rachel Haduch and Leslie Haduch

POSTURE AND BALANCE
EVEN BALANCE · HEEL LIFT · LEG BALANCE · PELVIC TILT · SITTING STRETCH · TOE TOUCH

INTERMEDIATE POSTURE
ROLLING POSTURE · REACHING STRETCH · ARM WINDOWS · 12 O CLOCK ARM CLOCK

GENTLE WARM-UP
ARM LIFT · CAT COW · HIP ROTATION · MARCHING · NECK ROTATIONS · NECK STRETCH · SHOULDER ROTATIONS · SPINAL ROTATIONS · TOE LIFTS · WRIST CIRCLES

INTERMEDIATE WARM-UP
PELVIC TILT · CLOCK EXERCISE

ARMS AND SHOULDERS
ARM LIFT · ARM REACH AND PULL · ARM REACH · HUG A TREE · PELVIC DROP · SHOULDER MOBILITY · SHOULDER STRETCH

INTERMEDIATE UPPER BODY
PUSH UP · ROW THE BOAT

STRENGTH IN THE CORE
CORE TURN · LEG LIFT · MOUNTAIN CLIMBER · SIDE BEND · WALL PLANK

INTERMEDIATE UPPER BODY
CRUNCH WITH KNEE PULLS · CRUNCHES · SPINAL STRETCH · WALL BRIDGE

LOWER BODY ENDURANCE
CALF STRETCH · FORWARD LEG LIFT · HEEL SQUAT · KNEE BENDS · LUNGE · MINI SQUAT · SIDE LEG LIFT · SIDE STEP

INTERMEDIATE LOWER BODY
BACK LEG LIFTS · LITTLE LEG LIFT · WALL SIT

LOWER BODY ENDURANCE IN THE COOL DOWN
ANKLE CIRCLES · ARM AND WRIST · CHEST STRETCH · HAMSTRING STRETCH · HIP FLEXOR · HIP OPENER · HIP TWIST · TRICEPS STRETCH

INTRODUCTION

EMBRACING WELLNESS AND VITALITY IN THE SENIOR YEARS

My mother, Leslie, has turned back the wheel of time. Her body is toned and muscular. Her energy levels are through the roof. She has taken to waking up early in the morning and craving the endorphins she receives from exercising. She is a living success story of how transformative stretching and strengthening can be if practiced every week. Her dedication to her health and wellness has inspired me to prioritize fitness in my life and write this book to help others obtain the same level of vibrancy in their life that I see in her spirit. She is an encouragement to the power of the mind when we set our goals on creating a better life for ourselves.

Aging is a natural process of living, and we all experience the effects on our bodies as we grow older. We may not be able to stop the hands of time, but we may be able to slow them down. This book will guide you to setting your body up for success in healthy living so you can enjoy your golden years and love your body.

Pilates, originally called "Contrology," is a technique created by Joseph Pilates in the 1920s and it is still relevant today. "Contrology is complete coordination of body, mind, and spirit designed to give you suppleness, natural grace, and skill that will be unmistakably reflected in the way you walk, in the way you play, and in the way you work. You will develop muscular power with corresponding endurance, ability to perform arduous duties, to play strenuous games, to walk, run or travel for long distances without undue body fatigue or mental strain."(Pilates, 1945)

Joseph Pilates was a success story in his own right. Throughout his childhood, he suffered from various ailments that affected his body and weakened his muscles, including rickets and rheumatic fever. These illnesses did not dampen his determination because he went on to become a successful gymnast, boxer, and circus performer.

Joseph Pilates observed that if an area of the body were misaligned, our muscles and joints would overcompensate, often resulting in injuries. He realized the importance of posture and balance within the body for a successful fitness program. In the 1920s, he owned a studio above the New York City Ballet. He instructed many actors, gymnasts, and athletes in developing core strength, often rehabilitating those affected by injury. He is known to have worked with many celebrities, including Katherine Hepburn!

After his death at 83 from Emphysema, his wife Clara continued teaching the Pilates method and began to teach apprentices so that these methods could be utilized by all who needed them. Often referred to as the 'Pilates Elders,' many of these Pilates instructors went on to live long and healthy lives, including his wife Clara, who lived to 94. She claims never to have contracted arthritis or any degenerative disease and continued to exercise into her 90s. Clara observed that most Americans use only about 10% of their muscles daily, leading to muscle atrophy and body pain in the later years. (Rhinebeck Pilates.) Most sports (besides swimming) also do not focus on all muscle groups and do not tone the whole body.

Our goal in this program is to find balance in our bodies, to empower our motivation, and to enhance the vitality of the spirit. We see this newly developed practice of Wall Pilates as a gentle way to find the results Joseph Pilates aimed for with his exercise regimen. This program varies slightly from the traditional mat Pilates because it uses the body's weight to increase balance, posture, and stamina. Wall Pilates makes exercise for Seniors easily accessible, and it's possible to increase resistance as you continue to challenge yourself.

Do you want more stamina and mobility?

Practice the exercises in this book, and you can feel more confident in your abilities.

Are you ready to take up a physical hobby that benefits your body?

This book will encourage you to meet your goals and get you excited about exercise!

Successful aging means making lifestyle choices that benefit your health, so that "Old in Years" becomes your "Golden Years!"

If we embrace life instead of dreading it, we can thrive. As we grow in years, we must continue to tone our bodies to remain flexible, and our self-confidence in our abilities stays strong. We can be our best selves if we continue working on our coordination, balance, and strength. The practices outlined in this book are a guide to achieving the wellness and vitality possible for any person of any age to reach.

1

THE FOUNDATIONS OF WALL PILATES

Congratulations on Starting Your Journey to Improved Mobility!

Imagine standing at the shore of a vast ocean, ready to embark on a journey of transformation and health. The first few times you swim out to sea, you test the waters and can only go so far. As you practice your strokes and strengthen your body, you become more confident and toned. Your body feels strong, and your mind feels calm and confident. This chapter begins the journey, equipping you with the tools to step into the sea of wellness potential that is your future.

Like the full-body workout that swimming can provide, Wall Pilates is also a full-body routine, with the added benefit that you don't have to leave your home! It takes 10-15 minutes a day to start feeling the effects of this balancing and energizing practice.

This form of exercise is perfect for Seniors in numerous ways. Wall Pilates has a reduced risk of injury because it focuses on controlled, low-impact movements. We utilize the wall as a guide, helping individuals align their bodies correctly during the postures. The wall also absorbs some of the pressure of the exercise, which reduces the impact on the joints.

Flexibility is crucial for seniors to prevent injury and maintain a full range of motion. Wall Pilates includes stretches and movements that can improve our resilience over time. This type of exercise can also be adapted to accommodate various physical limitations or medical conditions that seniors may have. The wall Pilates exercises in this book are adaptable to individual needs and varying fitness levels.

For seniors with chronic pain conditions, Wall Pilates can offer gentle movement and stretches that may help alleviate discomfort over time. These exercises often mimic real-life movements, promoting functional fitness. Wall Pilates can help seniors perform everyday activities with greater ease and confidence.

Pilates doesn't just positively influence the body; it also has many positive impacts on your mind such as promoting mental focus and mindfulness during exercise, which can help improve coordination and cognitive function. We must also strengthen the mind to create a workout practice that we know and love to do. To boost our self-esteem, we will start our wall Pilates journey with gentle movements and work up to challenging postures.

Simple movements may become more difficult as we age, but this doesn't mean we should accept this as usual. We are responsible for caring for this precious body we are gifted with. Many are put off by exercise because they feel it may be too strenuous or challenging. We are bringing Wall Pilates to you through this easy-to-follow format. In this book, you'll see how simple it is to establish a gentle yet effective practice.

Some may believe that Wall Pilates is not a form of strength training because it does not use external resistance or weights. Although Pilates is not explicitly designed to build muscle, it does build strength in all areas of the body, not just a few targeted muscle groups. This exercise gives the body all-around muscle strength that enhances mobility.

"Pilates is a whole-body workout that builds strength as well as balanced mobility and stability through all the joints in the body. So, you are not only controlling the movement against the wall resistance, but you are also moving through various planes of motion and ranges." (Economou, 2022)

We will be emphasizing the importance of safety as we teach the exercises. Compared to other fitness styles, there is a low risk of injury with wall Pilates. It can be very gentle on the body if done correctly and with care. We will guide you in navigating these postures in the safest way possible.

A study in the *Journal of Sports Science and Medicine* found that women over 65 who practiced Pilates for one hour three times per week over 12 weeks improved their flexibility and balance and decreased the number of falls in these women. (Babayigit, 2011) This study proves how valuable this practice can be for gaining independence, feeling safer in your body, and having confidence as you age. We will continue to build on these basics to obtain lasting results.

INSPIRING SENIOR BIO: FLO MEILER

As someone who loves a challenge, Flo Meiler has asserted herself as a winner in the world of Track and Field. At 60 years old, she began competing in many areas on the track, including high jump, long jump, hurdles, weight throw, and javelin. When she turned 65, she became interested in pole vaulting, which she loves because it is challenging.

Flo trains five days a week to keep her body in shape. She travels around the country, competing in the senior games and internationally on Team USA. Now, at 85, she continues to bring home medals and break records, inspiring others to follow their dreams for the love of the challenge. According to Flo, "If you don't use it, you lose it." (Weisholtz, 2019).

2

CREATING A SAFE SPACE FOR YOUR WALL PILATES PRACTICE

 "A healthy body is a platform for a healthy mind to flourish."

— *PAWAN MISHRA*

SETTING THE MOOD

As we delve deeper into the world of Wall Pilates for seniors, it's crucial to emphasize the importance of having a safe and comfortable environment for your practice. Creating a suitable space in your home can enhance your Wall Pilates experience, making it more enjoyable and conducive to achieving your fitness goals. This chapter will explore the steps and considerations for setting up a space that promotes safety, comfort, and optimal results for your Wall Pilates journey.

Start by choosing a location that is quiet and calm. A peaceful environment allows for relaxation and deeper concentration. Make a consistent time 3-4 times a week of 10-15 minutes during the day to successfully work exercise into your daily routine. Consider beginning your day with this practice to wake your brain and body up.

Minimize distractions by choosing a time to exercise that you will not be interrupted. Choose a space where no other people are walking through or talking. Also, turn off any devices that may become bothersome.

Give yourself ample space to move during your wall Pilates practice. Clear any clutter or obstacles out of the way so that you have about a 10x10 ft area against the wall where you can stretch out. Wear clothing that is form-fitting and comfortable.

Use a sturdy, strong wall that can safely hold your weight. Make sure nothing is hanging that may get in your way as you are leaning or holding onto the wall.

The floor must have a non-slip surface so that no injuries occur. We recommend a yoga mat for floor exercises, so you do not slip. Practicing your workouts on a carpet can also give you the traction you need for proper posture. Good lighting and a comfortable temperature will also create a safe space to practice Wall Pilates.

Wall Pilates does not require expensive equipment, making it easily accessible at home and at your convenience. All the equipment listed is optional. A yoga mat can help with creating a safe floor area to work on. Cushions or yoga blocks can provide comfort and support when stabilizing the body in a deep pose. A chair is optional as an additional support and aid in many postures. Also, weights are suggested in some of the postures if you want more of a challenge.

Creating an inviting mood can obtain the serene atmosphere we want during Pilates. Putting on some soothing music can help the body relax into the postures. Personalize your space by putting a picture of a loved one, a picture of a destination you are traveling to that you want to be fit for, or an affirmation you resonate with. These reminders can inspire you to be the best version of yourself.

TIPS TO PRIORITIZE SAFETY

- Take precautions to prevent any injuries.
- Start with gentle movements and gradually increase the Range of Motion. Listen to your body to avoid any strain or discomfort.
- Maintain proper posture and alignment throughout the exercise. Remember to rely on the wall for that increased support.
- Remember to always hydrate with lots of water before exercising! Bring it with you to your practice so that you have it readily available. Drink lots of water after you finish your Wall Pilates so your muscles can recover optimally.

Creating a safe and comfortable space for Wall Pilates in your home is essential in your journey to improved health and fitness as a senior. By carefully selecting the location, prioritizing safety, and setting the right mood, you'll be well-prepared to enjoy the benefits of Wall Pilates in a space that promotes relaxation and focus. Remember that your Wall Pilates space should reflect your unique preferences and needs, providing a haven for physical and mental well-being.

INSPIRING SENIOR BIO: YUICHIRO MIURA

Summiting Mount Everest is an achievement many people cannot imagine conquering. Yuichiro Miura became the oldest person in the world to summit Mt. Everest in May of 2013 at the age of 80. Many people have died trying to summit Everest, yet this Japanese alpinist has summited it three times, all over the age of 70! Yuichiro also underwent four heart surgeries before his last summit, making his achievement more awe-inspiring. He says, "You need a target, no matter how big or small, and to build your health and fitness towards it." (Goldfarb, 2018) This elder shows that creating goals for our health journey helps to manifest the outcome we are working towards.

3

MASTERING PROPER BREATHING TECHNIQUES

 "Above all, learn how to breathe correctly."

— *JOSEPH PILATES*

Breathing is a fundamental need of our existence, an involuntary action often unnoticed on the daily. Yet, when it comes to practicing Wall Pilates, how we breathe becomes a powerful tool that can significantly impact our overall performance, comfort, and success in achieving our fitness goals. This chapter delves into mastering breathing techniques tailored to seniors engaged in Wall Pilates.

For many seniors, Wall Pilates is an incredible avenue to improve strength, flexibility, and balance while promoting a sense of mental clarity and well-being. However, the depth of these benefits can be unlocked and amplified through the conscious and deliberate application of proper breathing techniques.

BENEFITS OF PROPER BREATHING

Proper breathing enhances the effectiveness of exercises including:

1. Improved muscle function and precision.
2. Improved core engagement and stability.
3. Increase in oxygen.
4. Reduced blood pressure and heart rate.
5. Reduced risk of injury.
6. Reduced muscle tension.
7. Increased mind-body connection.

DIAPHRAGMATIC BREATHING

Also known as deep belly or abdominal breathing, this type of breathing is a fundamental technique that can enhance your Wall Pilates practice. It promotes relaxation, core stability, and efficient oxygen exchange.

Follow these step-by-step instructions to master diaphragmatic breathing:

1. Begin with Good Posture:

- Sit or stand with your spine aligned against the wall.
- Relax your shoulders, keeping them down and away from your ears.

- Place your feet hip-width apart for stability.

2. Inhale Slowly Through Your Nose:

- Take a slow, deep breath in through your nose.
- As you inhale, feel your abdomen expand and rise. Imagine filling a balloon in your belly.

3. Exhale Gradually Through Your Mouth:

- Exhale slowly and evenly through your mouth, allowing the air to flow naturally.
- Feel your abdomen gently contract and lower as you exhale.

4. Be Mindful of Your Breath:

- Focus on the rhythm of your breath.
- Inhale for a count of 5, and exhale for a count of 5.

5. Engage Your Diaphragm:

- As you breathe in, consciously engage your diaphragm, the muscle below your lungs. Feel it expand and contract with your breath.

6. Keep Chest Movement Minimal:

- Avoid excessive chest movement. The primary expansion and contraction should occur in your abdomen.

7. Maintain Relaxation:

- Ensure that you remain relaxed throughout the practice.
- Tension in your neck, shoulders, or jaw may indicate shallow breathing.

8. Repeat and Practice:

- Continue this diaphragmatic breathing pattern for 5-10 minutes.
- Gradually extend the duration as you become more comfortable.
- Incorporate diaphragmatic breathing at the beginning and end of your Wall Pilates practice and during challenging exercises to maintain composure and stability.

Following your breathing is the first way to create mindfulness in your Wall Pilates practice. Use this steady breathing exercise as an anchor in your movement. As you move, use nonjudgemental observation to recognize how you are experiencing the exercise in the present moment. Focus on the quality of each movement rather than the quantity of postures. Ultimately, the goal is to cultivate a sense of flow and grace.

INSPIRING SENIOR BIO: TAO PORCHON-LYNCH

Founder of the Westchester Institute of Yoga, this incredible woman has proven that age doesn't define our abilities. At 98, she is now in the Guinness Book of World Records as the World's oldest yoga teacher. She has taught for over 45 years and continues to teach multiple styles of yoga in Hartsdale, New York. She continues to drive and travel the world, teaching yoga workshops, and still loves wearing heels when she goes out! She is also the award-winning author of Dancing Light: The Spiritual Side of Being Through the Eyes of a Modern Yoga Master. She is living proof of her mantra, "There is nothing we can't do if we harness the power within us." (Blog, Yoga 2016)

4

BALANCE AND POSTURE ENHANCEMENT

"The Miracle isn't that I finished, the miracle is that I had the courage to start."

— *JOHN BINGHAM*

As we age, maintaining equilibrium becomes paramount for preventing falls and enhancing the overall quality of our daily activities. Wall Pilates offers a gentle yet practical approach to finding your center of gravity by improving balance and proper posture. Join us as we delve into the fundamental principles, exercises, and mindfulness practices guiding you toward renewed confidence and vitality.

PROPRIOCEPTION

Often referred to as the body's "sixth sense," proprioception plays a pivotal role in achieving and maintaining balance. It is the intricate ability of our body to sense its position in space and respond to changes in our environment without conscious thought. For our equilibrium, proprioception allows us to make subtle adjustments in muscle tension and joint angles to remain steady on our feet. This innate sense helps us understand where our body parts are in relation to one another and the environment, enabling us to adapt swiftly to changes in terrain, posture, or weight distribution. In the practice of Wall Pilates, becoming aware of our proprioception is a crucial element in enhancing physical stability, confidence, and overall well-being.

POSTURE CHECK

To improve our proprioception and develop better balance, we can use specific exercises that challenge our body's ability to adapt. First, we must determine how aligned our body is by doing a posture check. While standing tall in front of the mirror, ask yourself the following questions:

- Does your head tilt to one side?
- Are your shoulders and hips level?
- Is your weight evenly distributed?
- Does your back arch?
- Does your chin jut out?

Now, to realign your posture:

- Use non-judgmental observation of your alignment.
- Face the mirror with your feet facing forward and directly below your hips.
- Distribute your weight evenly.
- Stack your knees above your ankles.
- Set hips above your knees.
- Lengthen your spine, imagining you have a bunch of helium balloons tied to the top of your head, lifting you taller.
- Relax your neck and jaw.
- Notice the changes and how you feel different.

PERSONALIZE YOUR PRACTICE

Every individual has varying abilities of strength, flexibility, and mobility. We encourage each person to do what is best for their own body. Many of these exercises will have modifications to make them easier or harder based on your ability. Listen to your body to determine what is best for you.

Basic Exercises are accessible to the most beginner in the Wall Pilates practice. We encourage you to ensure you feel confident in the Basic Exercises before trying the Intermediate practices. Intermediate exercises require sitting or lying on the ground or are particularly challenging.

The more you work these exercises into your daily life, the more you will develop muscle memory for maintaining the proper posture and balance. To cultivate mindful posture throughout the day, incorporate it into your daily activities.

BASIC WALL POSTURE EXERCISES

The goal is to feel balanced and comfortable in our bodies, beginning with our alignment. We will now continue with exercises that can benefit your posture in the long run. These are easy exercises that challenge our posture so that we can be aware of our everyday alignment.

EVEN BALANCE

Bring awareness to how you are distributing your weight.

1. Stand up straight and tall with your arms hanging loose by your sides.

2. Soften your gaze and bring your attention to your feet and toes.

3. Focus on bearing your weight evenly between your feet.

4. Balance each foot's weight between the heels, the big toes, and the middle toes.

5. Imagine rooting down to the earth's center, cultivating balance and sturdiness.

6. Keep your joints loose, avoiding locking your knees.

7. Now, lengthen your spine so that an opposite force then gravity works in your movement.

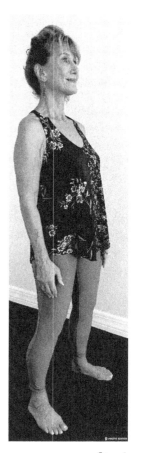

Step 1

WALL TOE TOUCHES

Strengthen your inner balance.

1. Stand tall with your left hand on the wall and your body at a right angle with the wall.

2. Move your right foot back to balance on your toes on that foot. Keep both legs straight but joints unlocked.

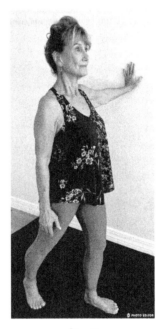

Step 2

3. Challenge Yourself:

- Remove your hand from the wall.
- Move your head up and down and left and right while balancing.

PELVIC TILT

An exercise that brings awareness to the posture and spinal alignment.

1. Stand up straight and tall with your hands on your hips.

2. Isolate the rotation of the hips by tilting the pelvis forward while keeping the chest, back, and legs still.

3. Rotate the hips back, feeling the lower back curve, and straighten.

4. Repeat this forward and backward movement ten times.

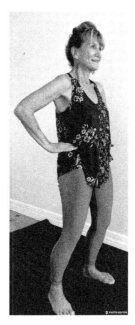

Step 2

SITTING STRETCH

A way to feel your posture against the support of the wall.

1. Sit with your spine straight and tall with your back and hips against the wall and your shoulders relaxed. If you have trouble sitting on the ground, you can do this exercise in a chair.

2. Legs are extended straight out in front of you with a slight bend in the knee if needed.

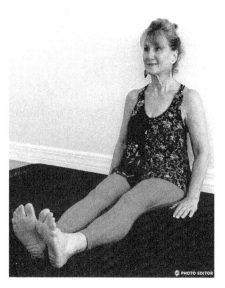

Step 2

3. Flex your feet and press your back, shoulders, and head into the wall.

4. Take 5 deep breaths in through the nose and out through the mouth.

WALL HEEL LIFTS

A calf strengthening and balancing exercise.

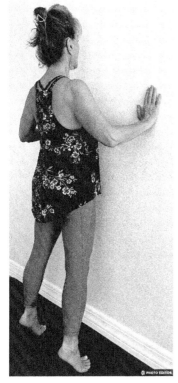

Step 3

1. Stand facing the wall with your feet shoulder-width apart and your hands on the wall.

2. Lengthen your spine and relax your shoulders.

3. Inhale as you raise onto your toes, leaning forward towards the wall. To reduce the intensity of the stretch, you can lift one heel at a time.

4. Exhale as you come back onto your heels.

5. Repeat 10 times, following the breath with your movements.

6. Challenge Yourself:

- Hold the Heel Lift for the count of 3.
- See if you can lift your hand off the wall to practice balancing.

WALL-ASSISTED LEG BALANCE

Enhances balance, posture, and lower body strength and stability.

1. Start with the wall at your side, holding it with your left hand.

- Some may also like a chair to hold onto for support.

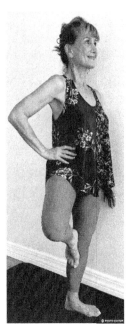

2. Lift the right leg off the ground and place the bottom of your foot on your ankle with your toe pointing towards the ground.

3. Hold the pose for the count of 5.

4. Continue with the right side of the body.

5. Challenge yourself:

Step 2

- To let go of the wall to find your balance.
- Place the raised leg on the inside of your calf.

INTERMEDIATE WALL POSTURE EXERCISES

ARM WINDOWS

This stretch brings awareness to the spine and strength to the arms.

1. Sit with your back and hips against the wall with your legs extended straight out in front of you.

2. As you inhale, bring your arms up in front of you, so that they are parallel to the floor.

- Palms facing down.

3. As you exhale, Slide your elbows back toward the wall, keeping your forearm parallel to the ground. Your arm is now at a 90-degree angle with your elbows sticking out from your body.

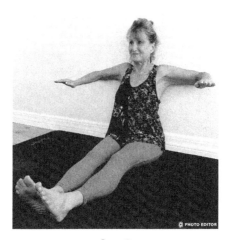

Step 3

4. On the inhale, raise your forearm against the wall with your arm still at a 90-degree angle. Your palms are facing away from the wall.

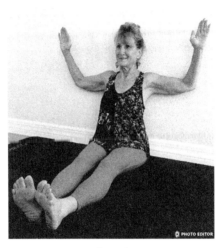

Step 4

5. On the exhale, raise your arms up and over your head. - Try to keep your arms as close to the wall as possible.

6. Now, let's reverse the exercise. On the inhale, drop your elbows so that your arms are at a 90-degree angle against the wall.

- Your forearms are touching the wall.

7. On the exhale, drop your forearms parallel to the floor, keeping the arms at a 90-degree angle.

8. On the inhale, bring your arms straight out in front of you.

9. Repeat the exercise 5 times.

REACHING STRETCH

Feeling the strength and length of the spine.

1. Sit with your back and hips against the wall. If sitting on the floor is too challenging, you can do this exercise in a chair.

2. Extend your legs straight out in front of you. Put a slight bend in your knees if necessary and flex your feet.

3. Inhale and raise your arms up and over your head against the wall.

4. As you exhale, forward fold down towards your knees, keeping your arms straight as you reach past your feet. Hold for the count of 10.

Keep your lower back against the wall, pulling your belly button towards your spine.

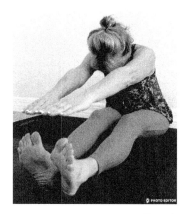

Step 4.

WALL ARM CLOCK

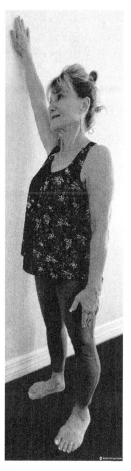

Step 6

Focus on keeping the shoulders square with the hips while allowing the spine to elongate.

1. Stand up straight with your right shoulder almost touching the wall. Step away from the wall to reduce the intensity of the stretch.

2. Place your feet shoulder-width apart. Align your posture so that your spine feels straight and long.

3. Your arm will be the hour hand on your wall clock. You start at 6 o'clock with your arm at your side and your palm against the side of the wall.

4. Now rotate your arm up to 9 o'clock with a straight arm.

5. Hold each position to the count of three breaths. Take a breath through the nose, inflating your diaphragm, then release the breath. Keep your other arm by your side.

6. Move your arm up to the 12 o'clock position and take 3 breaths.

7. Move your arm to the 1 o'clock position, keeping your arm as straight as possible and take 3 breaths.

8. As you move your arm from the 1 o'clock position to the 3 o'clock position, focus on lengthening your spine and keeping your chest facing forward. Take 3 breaths.

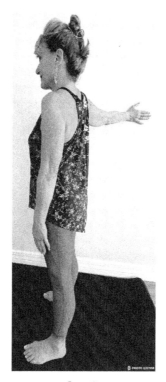

Step 8.

9. Face the opposite direction and repeat the stretch with the other arm.

ROLLING POSTURE EXERCISE

Stretch the spine and roll out tension in the vertebrae.

1. Lay with your back flat on the ground.

2. Hold your hands behind your knees and bring them towards your chest.

3. Slowly rock back towards your neck and then shift weight down towards your hips. Concentrate on feeling each vertebrae touch the ground.

4. Repeat 5 times.

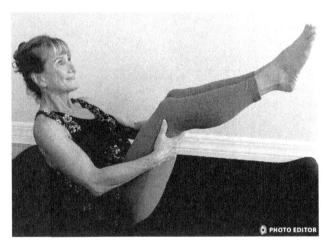

Step 2

DAILY POSTURE AWARENESS

- Have an awareness of your posture while sitting or standing.
- Use deep Breathing techniques to bring awareness to your body.
- Move around and exercise often.
- Make healthy choices to maintain a healthy weight.
- Wear comfortable shoes that offer support.
- Adjust your work environment to benefit your posture.

OVERCOMING CHALLENGES WITH WALL PILATES

The goal of this book is to create a Vibrant You. Whether your desire is to lose weight, become stronger, or feel more independent; we must overcome our obstacles and rise above challenges to grow. We will celebrate the resilience we create in our bodies and minds.

Sometimes, we must adapt our practice due to physical limitations. Throughout the book, modifications will be available to cater to many ability levels. We encourage you to listen to your body and challenge yourself to meet your personal fitness goals. If you have questions about any posture or practice, partner with your healthcare professional to ensure safe practice.

Before beginning this journey of self-improvement, I encourage you to sit down with a paper and pencil and outline your goals to get the most out of this book.

Ask yourself:

- What are my main goals? Weight Loss? Flexibility? Strength? Confidence? Body awareness?
- What physical limitations do I need to be aware of when exercising?
- How often do I want to exercise a week, and for how long?

Set a goal for yourself for how many weeks you can continue your practice. We have made it easy to stay motivated through our easy 21-day Wall Pilates Challenge at the end of this book. If you feel yourself going a week or even a month without meeting your goals, don't be too hard on yourself. Just come back to the practice and set new attainable goals to ensure you feel successful in your practice. Together, we will create the transformative power of perseverance.

INSPIRING SENIOR BIO: PAT GALLANTE-CHARETTE

Swimming is an incredible exercise for the whole body, but marathon swimming takes this exercise to the next level. At 65, Pat Gallante-Charette has excelled at this sport since she started at 50. It began when she completed an open ocean swimming marathon to honor her brother's life. Even though she had no prior experience, her determination and stamina kept her going. She is now working to complete the "Oceans Seven" challenge, which entails swimming seven of the longest open-water swims in the world. Even though she has struggled to meet this challenge with obstacles thwarting her swims, she says, " I could have thrown in the towel, but it actually strengthened my resolve." (Averill, 2022). This incredible dedication shows us how powerful the mind can be in overcoming life's challenges.

5

GENTLE WARM-UP AND FLEXIBILITY

"Take care of your body; it's the only place you have to live."

— *JIM ROHN*

P reparing Your Body for Movement is an essential step in your practice. We must start warming up the body and exploring its flexibility to ensure a safe and beneficial experience. In the warm-up, we focus on gentle, fluid movements to prepare the body for increasingly challenging postures. We will start with the neck and work down the body to relax our muscles and joints and boost circulation from the head to the feet.

BASIC WARM-UP EXERCISES

The following exercises help to slowly wake up your muscles to the incredible benefits of our Wall Pilates practice. You may feel new sensations in muscles that have been dormant. These warm-up exercises ensure a gentle awakening so that we start safely and with awareness of the body's abilities. Make sure you feel confident in your ability to do the basic warm-ups listed before moving on to the intermediate exercises.

NECK STRETCH

Loosen the muscles in the neck and release tension in the head and down through the spine.

1. Sit on the floor in a comfortable crossed-legged position or sit in a chair with your feet flat on the floor in front of you.

2. Place your hands behind your head with your palms touching the back of your head and interlace your fingers.

3. Gently use the weight of your arms and hands to tip your head and neck forward.

4. Count to 10, and then release your hands, allow your head to come back up to neutral, and then fall backward so that you look up at the ceiling.

5. Repeat this exercise 2 more times.

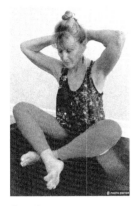

Step 3

NECK ROTATIONS

Relax the muscles at the base of the spine and down through the shoulders.

1. Start by standing tall with your shoulders pulled down and back, opening the chest.

- One hand may want to hold the wall or the back of a chair for added support.

2. Tip your head to the right side so your ear moves towards your right shoulder.

- Keep your shoulders down.
- Hold this position to the count of 5.

3. Roll your head forward so that your chin is resting towards your chest.

- Hold to the count of 5.

4. Tip your head to the left side so your ear moves towards your left shoulder.

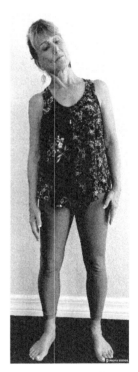

Step 2

- Your shoulders are relaxed down your back as you count to 5.

5. Roll your head back to look up at the ceiling and hold for the count of 5.

6. Continue this stretch 2 more times.

7. Challenge Yourself:

- Add a deeper stretch by gently holding your head above your ear with the arm your head tilts towards.

SHOULDER ROTATIONS

Realigning the posture and loosening the muscles in the neck and shoulders. Good practice in connecting the movement and the breath.

1. Stand in a relaxed posture with your arms by your sides.

- Relax your jaw and become aware of your breath.

2. As you inhale, bring your shoulders up towards your ears.

3. Slowly exhale, squeezing your shoulder blades towards your spine and dropping your shoulders down and away from your head.

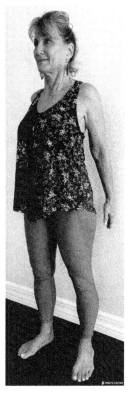

Step 3

4. End the motion with your shoulders relaxed and your neck feeling lengthened.

5. Repeat this exercise 5 times.

SPINAL ROTATIONS

Release tension around the spine and shoulders.

1. Sit on the floor with your legs straight out in front of you.

- Put a slight bend in your knee.
- This exercise can also be practiced seated in a chair with feet flat on the floor and shoulder-width apart.

2. Sit up straight with your shoulders relaxed.

3. Place your hands on your sternum with your fingers touching and elbows relaxed.

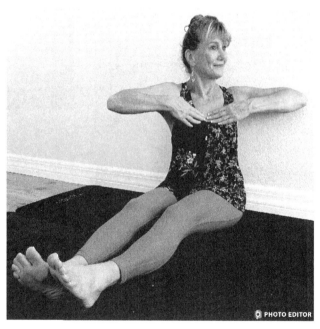

Step 3.

4. Take an inhale, and as you exhale, rotate around the spine to the left side.

- It should feel like you are drawing your left rib cage back and your right rib cage forward. Your arms and head should not be moving, only your rib cage.

5. Take a breath in this position.

6. Then, take another inhale and, on the exhale, rotate back to face forward.

7. Inhale and rotate right, taking another breath while facing right.

8. Continue for 8 more rotations.

WRIST CIRCLES

Increase mobility and flexibility in your wrists and arms.

1. Sit or stand with a straight spine and shoulders relaxed.

2. Hold your right forearm to steady your wrist.

3. Rotate your right hand clockwise 10 rotations and counter-clockwise 10 rotations.

4. Open and close your hand 5 times to stretch out your fingers.

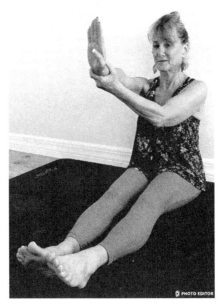

Step 4

5. Repeat with the other wrist.

ARM LIFTS

Strengthen and tone the arms and shoulders.

1. Stand with your feet shoulder-width apart and your arms by your sides.

2. On your inhale, lift your arms to shoulder height so that your hands point in opposite directions.

3. On the exhale, release your arms slowly down to your sides.

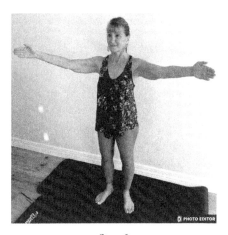

Step 3

4. Repeat 10 times.

5. Challenge Yourself:

- Hold the arm lift for 3-10 seconds.
- Use 2 lb. weights for added toning.

KNEE LIFTS

Assist with knee mobility and Range of Motion through marching.

1. Start by standing tall with your left hand on the wall next to you.

2. On the inhale, pick up one knee so it is just below hip height and hold for 3 seconds.

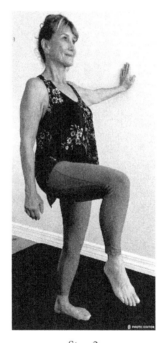

Step 2

3. Exhale and lower foot back to the ground.

4. Continue alternating each knee for a total of 10 knee lifts.

HIP OPENER ROTATIONS

Activates abdominal muscles and mobilizes the spine, stretching the hips and thighs.

1. Stand with feet shoulder-width apart next to a support such as a wall.

2. While holding on to the support with the left hand, lift your right knee in front of you so it is just below the level of your hips. Keep the left knee relaxed.

3. Open your hips by moving your right knee out to the right, down, and around, circling your knee in as large a circle as possible in the clockwise direction.

4. Continue for 5 complete hip opening circles, then switch to the other leg.

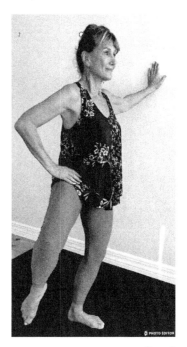

Step 2

TOE LIFTS

Challenge your balance and strengthen the lower legs.

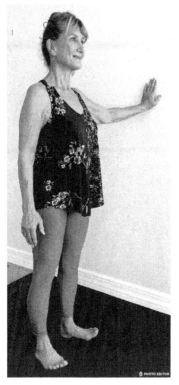

1. Stand with your feet together and arms relaxed. Place your hand on the wall for additional support.

2. Inhale as you lift your toes off the ground, ensuring the rest of your body stays in the same position.

3. Exhale as you lower your toes to the floor.

4. Continue 10 times.

Step 3

WALL CAT-COW

Stretch the back and neck.

1. Begin by placing your hands at shoulder height on your wall.

2. On your exhale, drop your head to look down at your toes. Relax your neck and shoulders.

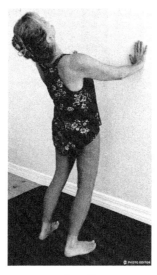

Step 2

3. On the inhale, lift your chest and head to stretch the neck and spine so that you are looking at the ceiling.

4. Continue to curl and round down on the exhale and arch to look up on the inhale for 10 repetitions.

INTERMEDIATE WARM-UP

When ready to take your warm-up to the next level.

TABLE-TOP PELVIC TILTS

Supports pelvic position and alignment.

1. Start by laying on the floor with your feet on the wall so your legs are at a 90-degree angle.

2. Tilt your pelvis up and back without lifting your back from the ground.

- The wall is an excellent support in this position to help with pelvic alignment.

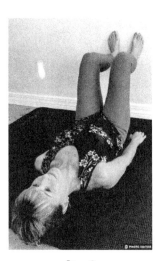

Step 2

CLOCK EXERCISE

Spine flexibility and pelvic alignment.

1. Start with your spine straight and your feet shoulder-width apart.

2. Put your hands on your hips to feel the movement of the pelvic rotation.

3. Tilt your pelvis in a circular movement as if 12 o'clock was above your navel, 6 o'clock was at the pelvic bone, and 3 and 9 o'clock were at each hip. Rotate around in a circle, feeling the fluid motion of your hips and pelvis swirling around.

4. Continue for 10 rotations.

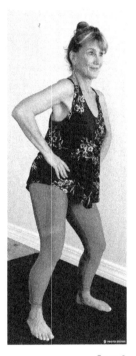

Step 3

INSPIRING SENIOR BIO: BETTY GOEDHART

We have all admired the skill and bravery required when watching trapeze artists swinging from up high. Betty Goedhart proves there is always time to pick up an athletic venture, even trapeze flying! She had always wanted to explore the trapeze. The first time she tried it, she was frightened when she reached the top of the ladder and looked down. she stated, "I knew I had to do it because I might never have another chance."

At 86 years old, Betty takes classes 4 times a week and participates in performances throughout the year. Her favorite move is the "razzle-dazzle," which involves leaping off the platform, turning around on the bar, swinging back and forth, and then letting go with a front flip into the safety net. Surprisingly she says, "It's an easy one I don't have to worry about, so I can smile the whole way through!" (Crouch, 2019). Betty proves you can do whatever you set your heart and mind on.

6

FOCUSING ON ARMS AND SHOULDERS

 "Age is whatever you think it is; You are as old as you think you are."

— *MUHAMMED ALI*

I applaud you on staying committed to a better you! These new feelings of strength and power within the body motivate many to continue toward increased mobility, independence, and confidence.

As we age there is a tendency for a natural loss of strength and muscle mass, particularly in the upper body. Wall Pilates is a vital tool in counteracting this decline by targeting certain muscle groups. When we tone our arms, shoulders and upper back we ensure our bodies continued capabilities.

These movements are building on the innate power we all have within us. As you grow more confident, we will explore the movements that can enable us to expand our Range of Motion and enhance our upper body strength.

BASIC ARM AND SHOULDER EXERCISES

These postures are essential for supporting everyday activities such as lifting objects or reaching to take something down from a high shelf.

We will begin with easy arm exercises that are specifically designed for safe use by Seniors and make upper body exercise convenient and accessible.

Listen to your body. When you are confident with your abilities you can work into more challenging postures.

ARM REACH

Shoulder flexibility and arm strength

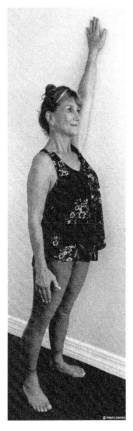

1. Start with your left shoulder about six inches from the wall.

2. Raise your arm to reach up the wall, as close to parallel with your ear as possible. Place your palm on the wall.

3. Continue to the count of 10 on the left side.

4. Turn so that your right side faces the wall and continue for the count of 10 on the right side.

Step 2

HUG A TREE

Develops upper body stability and shoulder strength.

1. Begin with your arms raised at shoulder height in front of you. Round your arms as if you were hugging a big tree.

2. Inhale as you draw your arms together as if closing your arms around the tree.

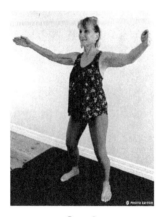

Step 2

3. Exhale as you open your arms wide.

- Pull your shoulder blades toward each other with your elbows facing the back of the room.

4. Continue this exercise for 10 repetitions.

5. Challenge Yourself:

- Do this exercise with weights for an added challenge.

SHOULDER MOBILITY EXERCISE

Stretching the shoulders and upper back.

1. Stand with your back against the wall and your feet shoulder-width apart.

2. As you inhale, lift your arms by your sides up over your head as high as possible so your arms are ideally against the wall.

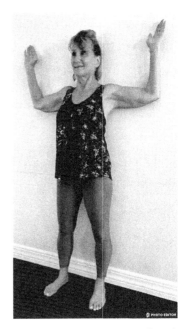

Step 1

- Move your arms as far back towards the wall as is comfortable.

3. As you exhale, bring your arms down along the wall into the "goal post" position.

- The "goal post" position means your elbows are at 90-degree angles.

4. Continue this stretch for a total of 10 repetitions.

PELVIC DROP

Opens the chest and strengthens the shoulders.

1. Stand with your back and your palms on the wall behind you.

2. Step away from the wall but keep your upper back against the wall.

3. Lift your pelvis so there is a straight line from your chest to your feet.

4. Inhale as you lower your pelvis so that it is pressed against the wall behind you.

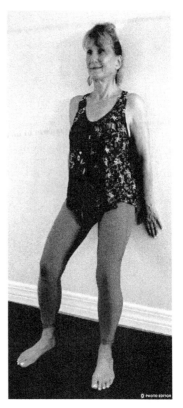

- Keep your arms and shoulders pressed against the wall so the pressure is held by the upper body.

Step 3. Step 4.

5. Exhale as you raise your pelvis again.

6. Continue for 10 repetitions.

ARM CIRCLES

Improve upper body ROM, develop coordination, and improve flexibility.

1. Begin standing with arms by your sides.

2. As you inhale, lift your arms in front of you as high as your shoulders.

- Aim to keep your fingers and arms straight and long.

3. Exhale as you open your arms wide into a v-position, keeping your arms in your peripheral vision to stay within the natural range of your shoulder joints.

4. Hold this position and take an Inhale.

5. Exhale as you bring your arms down to your sides.

6. Continue with 10 more repetitions of this exercise.

7. Challenge Yourself:

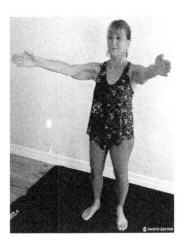

Step 3.

- Rotate arms in opposite direction for extra ROM support.
- Use 2 lb. weights to increase resistance.

SHOULDER STRETCH

Lengthen the spine and open the chest and shoulders.

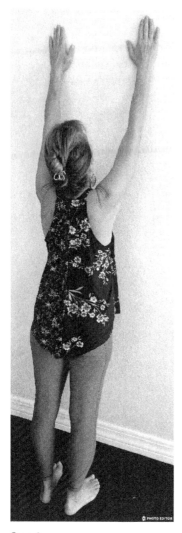

1. Start by standing facing the wall.

2. Reach above your head and touch the wall with your hands shoulder-width apart.

3. Step back from the wall and arch your back, stretching out the back and shoulders.

4. You can rest your forehead on the wall or look up towards the ceiling.

5. Continue to the count of 10.

Step 3

ARMS REACH AND PULL

Prepares the body for overhead work by strengthening arms and back.

1. Begin with hands behind your head and elbows out to the sides.

2. As you inhale, extend your arms up to the ceiling.

3. Keep your shoulder blades pulled down your back.

4. Exhale as you bend your elbows, and your hands move back behind your head to return to the starting position.

5. Repeat the exercise 10 times.

6. Challenge yourself:

- Perform single arm reach and pull by alternating one hand up at a time.
- Use 2 lb. weights for added toning.

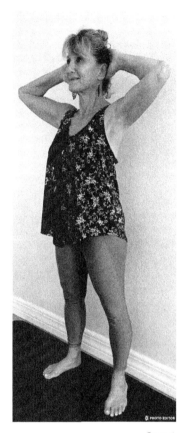

Step 1

INTERMEDIATE ARM AND SHOULDER EXERCISES

WALL PUSH-UPS

Increase arm strength and tone the core.

1. Begin by facing the wall with your feet shoulder-width apart.

2. Stand about 2 feet from the wall so you are not quite touching when you reach the wall.

3. Lean towards the wall and place your hands shoulder-width apart on the wall at shoulder height.

4. Tuck your tailbone in and envision a long, straight line running from your head down to the backs of your feet.

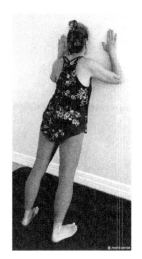

Step 5

5. Inhale as you bend your elbows and bring your face as close to the wall as possible. Trust your arms.

6. Exhale as you push out to lengthen your arms and feel your strength as you use your body as a natural weight.

7. Continue for a total of 10 wall push-ups.

8. Challenge Yourself:

- Step further away from the wall for an added stretch.

ROWING THE BOAT

Postures that benefit the arms, shoulders, and mid-back.

1. Begin seated with your legs in front of you in a slightly open V-position and your back against the wall.

- Practicing this position while seated in a chair can make this pose easier on the legs.

2. Bring your elbows out to the side with your thumbs near your chest.

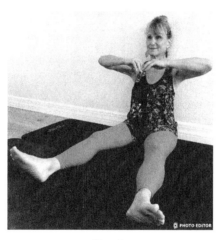

Step 2.

3. On the inhale, reach your arms up to the ceiling at a 45-degree angle.

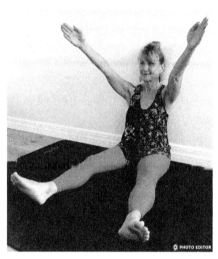

Step 3.

4. Slowly exhale as your arms draw a large semi-circle in the air, your fingers pointing in either direction, your fingers reaching, and your chest open.

5. Continue your exhale as you bring your hands back to the starting position with your thumbs by your chest.

6. Repeat these motions a total of 10 times.

7. Challenge Yourself:

- Do this exercise with 2 lb. weights in each hand.

INSPIRING SENIOR BIO: SISTER MADONNA BUDER

Sister Buder took up running at 50 from the suggestion of a priest to "harmonize mind, body and soul." This prompt opened a doorway for her of focus and fearlessness that led from running races to competing in over 400 triathlon competitions. Sister Madonna Buder has become known as the "Iron Nun," an endearing nickname for her incredible stamina as a triathlete.

She is the oldest woman to complete an Ironman Triathlon at the age of 82 and has continued to compete even at the age of 92. She states, "I love being outside in nature, and every time I'm tempted to discontinue competing, inspiring others keeps me going." (Fisher, 2022) She certainly is an inspiration with her sense of dedication. She proves that we can do hard things even into our later years.

Unlock the Power of Generosity

"Kindness is the sunshine in which virtue grows." - Robert Green Ingersoll

People who share kindness live fuller lives and radiate positivity. So, please take a moment to make a real difference.

Here's a simple question for you:

Would you extend a hand to someone you've never met, even if no one knew about it?

Imagine that person - it may be someone similar to you before you bought this book. Eager to make a positive change but still trying to figure out where to start. Our mission is to make Wall Pilates accessible to everyone, and your input is vital to achieving that mission.

This is where you play a crucial role. Most people do judge a book by its cover (and its reviews). So, I have a humble request on behalf of a fellow Senior you may never meet:

Please lend your voice to this cause by leaving a review for this book.

Your gift is free and takes less than a minute, yet it can reshape the life of a fellow senior. Your review might:

- *Enable a Senior to transform their life.*
- *Empower a person to be more confident in their body.*
- *Give hope to those who fear the journey.*
- *Make one more dream come true.*

To leave your review, scan the QR code below:

If the idea of anonymously helping a fellow senior appeals to you, welcome to the club. You're one of us.

I'm even more excited to share with you the strategies and insights that will help you enhance your life through Wall Pilates.

Thank you sincerely for your contribution. Now, let's get back to our journey.

Your biggest fans, [Rachel and Leslie Haduch]

PS - Did you know? Providing value to others makes you more valuable to them. If you think this book can help another senior, share it with them.

7

STRENGTH IN THE CORE, STRETCH IN THE SPINE

 "Every movement you do originates in the core."

— *SEAN VIGUE, PILATES FOR ATHLETES*

We all need a solid core to support our body through these exercises and into the world beyond our Wall Pilates practice. From simple movements such as walking, getting out of a chair, bending, or reaching; to more strenuous activities such as carrying heavy objects, we must strengthen our core for everyday use.

The core, comprising the abdomen, lower back, and pelvis muscles, plays a fundamental role in our daily activities and overall quality of life. In this context, core exercises for Seniors are significant to creating independence as we age.

BASIC CORE EXERCISES

We must build our core stability so that we can be strong like the trunk of a tree, providing balance and positive posture for the rest of the body. The exercises in this chapter offer many functional benefits to enhance overall vitality. These basic exercises are effective in alleviating pain in the back through healthy spinal movement.

Gradually progress from basic to intermediate exercises, that challenge and build your core and spine mobility, based on your personal progress and abilities.

WALL SIDE BEND

Stretch the spine and improve the posture.

1. Stand so that the wall is on your left side.

- Place your left hand on the wall to stabilize yourself during the stretch.

2. Cross your right leg in front of your left leg.

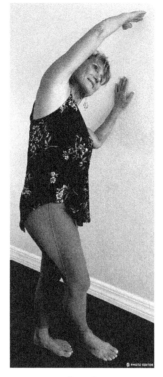

Step 3

3. Take a deep breath, and on the exhale, bring your right arm up and over your head, reaching towards the wall as far as possible.

4. Hold to the count of 10.

5. Repeat with the wall on your right side.

CORE TURN

Improve spine mobility, open the chest, and tone the core.

1. Start by facing the wall with your feet shoulder-width apart and about 2 ft from the wall.

- Keep your head, back, and legs in alignment.

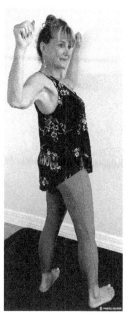

Step 3

2. Place your forearms on the wall with your hands in loose fists.

3. On the inhale, lift your right forearm off the wall and twist your ribcage, bringing your arm around your body, lifting, and opening your chest, and turning your head to the right.

4. Exhale and bring your arm back to the wall.

5. Alternate each side of the body by alternating your arms.

6. Continue with 10 repetitions on each side.

WALL PLANK

This pose is a full-body toning exercise that helps you gain confidence in your abilities.

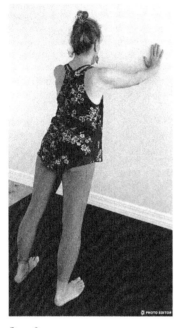

Step 3.

1. Begin by facing the wall with your feet shoulder-width apart.

2. Stand about 2 feet from the wall so you are not quite touching when you reach towards the wall.

3. Lean forward and place your hands shoulder-width apart on the wall with arms straight.

4. Tuck your tailbone in and envision a long, straight line running from your head down to the backs of your feet.

5. Hold this posture for the count of 10.

6. Challenge Yourself:

- Stand on the balls of your feet and walk farther from the wall to increase your body's angle from the wall. This angle increases the weight in your arms and is more work for your core and back.

WALL PLANK WITH LEG LIFTS

Challenge the glutes and core while stretching the shoulders and chest.

1. Begin by facing the wall in a Wall Plank position with your hands shoulder-width apart on the wall. Tuck your tailbone in and engage your core.

2. To initiate the movement, Inhale and extend your right leg out behind you, keeping it straight with your toes pointed.

3. Focus on keeping control of your movements by tightening the muscles in your glutes and core. Keep your eyes facing the wall.

4. Exhale and release your leg down.

5. Continue by alternating legs for a total of 10 repetitions on each side.

6. Challenge yourself:

- Lift your leg to shoulder height.

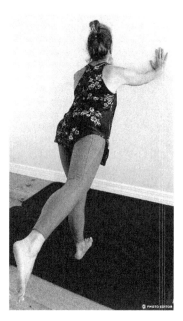

Step 2.

MOUNTAIN CLIMBER

Strengthen your back, tone your core, and mobilize your legs.

1. Begin in Wall Plank (Detailed Instructions on Page 67).

2. Stand about 2 feet from the wall and place your hands shoulder-width apart on the wall.

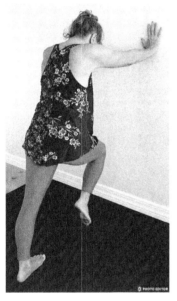

3. Tucking your tailbone in, take a step back so that you feel a stretch in the backs of your calves. You can come onto the balls of your feet to deepen the stretch.

4. Bring your knee towards your chest while bringing your head down towards your knee.

5. Alternate your knees for a total of 10 repetitions on each side.

Step 4.

INTERMEDIATE CORE EXERCISES

SPINAL STRETCH

Tighten the core and create elongation in the spine.

1. Begin by laying on your back with your feet flat on the ground and your knees together and take a deep breath in.

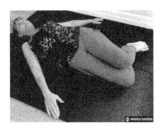

Step 2.

2. On your exhale, while stabilizing your torso with your palms on the ground, drop your knees to the left side, stacking your knees on top of each other as you bring them towards the floor. Turn your head to the right. Hold the stretch for the count of 3.

3. On the inhale, bring your knees back up to center with your feet once again flat on the ground.

4. On the exhale, drop your knees to the right side. Turn your head to the left. Release for a deep stretch in the hips and spine for a count of 3.

5. Continue alternating side to side for a total of 10 spinal stretches.

WALL BRIDGE

Improve hip stability while strengthening the glutes, hamstrings, and core.

1. Begin by lying on a non-slip surface with your feet on the wall so that your legs create a 90-degree angle at the knee. Your arms can rest by your sides with palms facing down.

2. Activate your core by drawing your naval down towards your spine.

3. As you inhale, press your feet into the wall, lift your hips, and lower back off the ground.

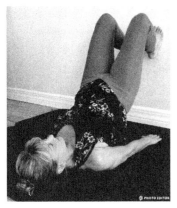

4. As you exhale, lower your back to the ground with controlled movement.

5. Repeat for a total of 5 wall bridges.

6. Challenge Yourself:

Step 3.

- You can alternately hold the wall bridge for 3-10 seconds.

TABLETOP WALL CRUNCHES

Build "six-pack" ab muscles and increase stability and strength.

1. Begin laying on the floor with feet on the wall and knees at a 90-degree angle.

2. Bend arms open and place hands on the sides of your head.

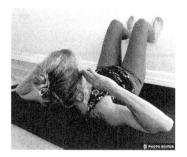

Step 3.

3. As you inhale, lift your head towards your knees to look at your belly button.

- Engage the core.
- Refrain from pulling your head up with your arms.
- Keep your arms open and relaxed.

4. As you exhale, tuck your chin, and release your head down to the mat.

5. Continue for 10 repetitions.

6. Challenge Yourself:

- Hold and twist left elbow to right knee, alternating to right elbow to left knee.

WALL CRUNCHES WITH KNEE PULLS

Build your core control and strength.

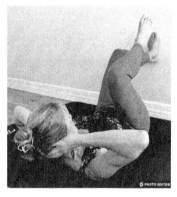

Step 3.

1. Lay on the floor with the bottoms of your feet on the wall so that your knees are at a 90-degree angle.

2. Place your hands under your head.

3. Bring the left knee up towards the head and the chin towards the knee.

- Engage your core and control the movements of your legs.

4. Continue for a total of 10 repetitions, alternating legs.

INSPIRING SENIOR BIO: HARRIET THOMPSON

At 94 years old, Harriet Thompson is one of the most senior women to have run a marathon. A two-time cancer survivor, Harriet has raised more than $100,000 for cancer research through the marathons she has run every year. Even though she took up running marathons at 76, it has never stopped her from working her hardest to complete such physically demanding goals. She is an avid Pilates practitioner and has used these exercises to help strengthen her body for the "long run."

Harriet has survived cancer and runs to benefit its research. Even though the physical challenges of battling cancer, she says she "still had the same incentive of trying to help, and the cancer just made it stronger. I realized what it was like to have cancer, and it made me want to give back more and to help this cause." It is inspiring to turn such a challenging experience into one that drives a person to create good for others. Harriet continues to inspire us after her passing with the notion that when things get tough, we say to ourselves, "This is a piece of cake. I can do this." (Butler, 2017).

8

LOWER BODY ENDURANCE BUILDING

As we age gracefully, our bodies undergo changes that impact our physical strength and overall mobility. One area of focus that often gets overlooked is strengthening the muscles in the lower body. These muscle groups, including quadriceps, hamstrings, and hip flexors, play a pivotal role in day-to-day activities such as climbing stairs, bending down, and walking. These Wall Pilates exercises help us maintain an active and independent lifestyle, especially as we age.

Strengthening our lower body can have a very beneficial impact to our joints in the hips, knees, and ankles by increasing circulation and decreasing joint stiffness. Wall Pilates promotes a supportive environment for joint health because of the low impact nature of the exercises. These exercises help maintain bone health through exercises that use our body weight or added weights to increase bone density and health.

BASIC LEG EXERCISES

These are our favorite leg workouts essential for beginner leg mobility. We are focusing on postures that are gentle yet effective at targeting age-related challenges, providing Seniors with a safe means of maintaining and improving their lower body function.

MINI SQUAT

Build more strength and mobility in your thighs and calves.

1. Begin with your back to the wall and your feet shoulder-width apart.

2. Your heels are about 4 inches from the wall, and your hands are on your hips.

3. Inhale and squat down so that your glutes touch the wall.

- Keep your chest lifted.
- Use the wall as a guide for how low to squat.
- Keep your weight over your feet.

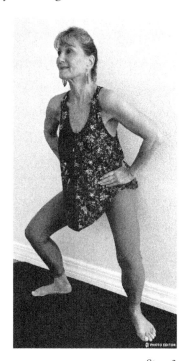

Step 3

4. Exhale and stand up.

5. Continue for 10 repetitions of this movement.

6. Challenge Yourself:

- Move farther away from the wall for a deeper squat.

WALL CALF STRETCH

A deep stretch in the side of your calf.

1. Start by facing the wall.

2. Step forward with your left foot and place your heel in front of the wall with your toes up on the wall.

3. Lean towards the wall to elongate the muscles in the calf and thigh.

4. Count to 10 for each side of the leg.

5. Release and point the toes.

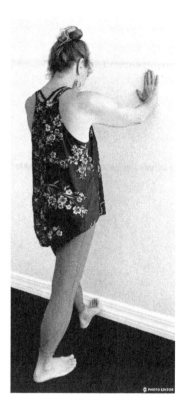

FORWARD WALL LUNGE

Calves get an excellent elongation, and thighs get tightened.

1. Begin by facing the wall with your palms on the wall in front of you.

2. Step back with your right leg on the inhale to feel a stretch in the calf.

- Keep your chest lifted.

3. On the exhale, step back to standing.

4. Continue for 10 repetitions on each side.

5. Challenge yourself:

- Step further back for a deeper stretch.

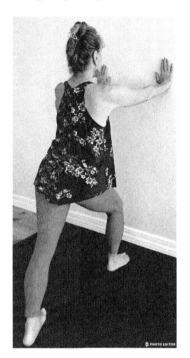

Step 3.

WALL HEEL SQUAT

Activating strength in the calf and thigh.

1. Start by facing the wall and holding it for support.

2. Create a slight bend in the knee with your feet facing out.

- Keep your posture tall.

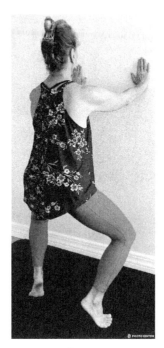

Step 2

3. Raise and lower your heels 10 times.

WALL FORWARD LEG LIFTS

Find mobility and strength in the thighs and glutes.

1. Hold onto the wall with your left hand.

2. Lift your right leg off the ground in front of you with your toes pointed to engage the entire leg.

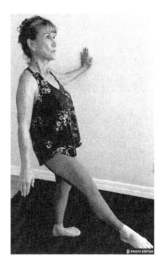

Step 3

- The leg standing can be slightly bent.
- Keep your hips even with the floor.

3. On the exhale, the toe touches the floor.

4. Repeat 10 times.

5. Challenge Yourself:

- Lift your leg as high as your hips.

WALL SIDE LEG LIFTS

A great outer thigh stretch.

1. Stand with both your hands supporting you on the wall.

2. On your inhale, lift your right leg off the ground to your side with your toes pointed.

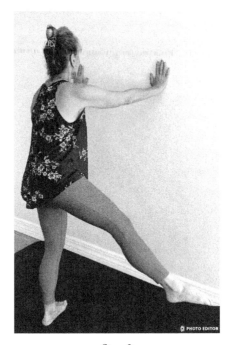

Step 2

3. On your exhale, lower your toe down to the ground.

4. Repeat on each side 5 times.

WALL KNEE BENDS

A challenge to stability and encourages a lengthened spine for better posture.

1. Stand tall with the wall on your left side and your feet together.

2. Inhale as you step back with your right foot.

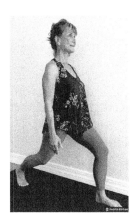

Step 2

- Redistribute your weight to center your upper body between your feet.

3. Exhale as you bend your knees, your back knee dropping towards the floor as far as you are comfortable.

- Keep your shoulders stacked on top of your hips to maintain good posture.
- The front foot should stay flat on the ground.

4. Exhale as you straighten both knees and push up with your back foot.

5. Repeat the motion 5 times on each side.

6. Challenge Yourself:

- Bring the back knee farther towards the floor.

WALL SIDESTEP

Increase your balance and tone the front of the legs.

1. Start with the wall close to your left side and your hand upon the wall.

2. On the inhale, Step out to your right side with your right leg.

3. Exhale and bend the knees in a slight squat.

4. Inhale and straighten the legs.

5. Exhale, bring your feet together.

6. Continue for 5 repetitions on each side.

7. Challenge Yourself:

• Deepen your squat.

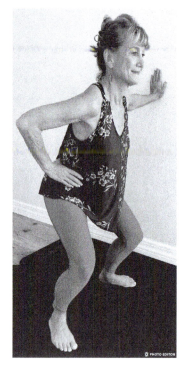

Step 3

INTERMEDIATE LEG EXERCISES

WALL LITTLE LEG LIFTS

Strength building for the whole leg.

1. Lay on your side with your head in your hand and the bottom of your feet against the wall.

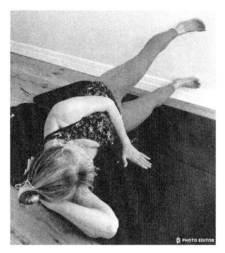

Step 3.

2. Lift your top leg comfortably, keeping your core engaged and flexing your feet.

3. Continue for 10 repetitions on each side of the body.

4. Challenge Yourself:

- Circle your upper leg around forwards and backward.

WALL BACK LEG LIFTS

A stretch to elongate the backs of the thighs.

1. Begin by laying on a mat with straight legs elevated a foot up the wall at a comfortable angle.

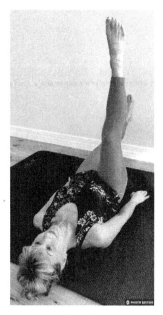

Step 2

2. Lift one leg at a time over your head as far as is comfortable.

3. Tap the wall with your foot and lift.

4. Continue for 10 total repetitions, alternating between legs.

WALL SIT

Tone the upper and lower legs and improve your balance.

1. Begin standing with your back to the wall.

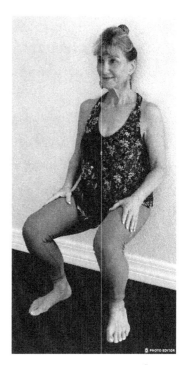

Step 2.

- Your heels should be about 6 inches from the wall and shoulder-width apart.

2. Lean back so that your back and head are against the wall.

3. Lower your back down the wall a few inches. You will begin to feel a stretch in your upper legs and calves.

4. Find a posture where you can endure the muscle burn and hold this for a count of 10.

5. Put your hands on the wall and step back to leave this position.

6. Continue for 3 repetitions.

7. Give yourself a gentle forward fold to inverse the stretch.

8. Challenge Yourself:

- The more parallel your thighs are to the ground, the harder this position will feel.

INSPIRING SENIOR BIO: ERNESTINE SHEPHERD

Exercise is a gateway to enhanced confidence and health, and we can begin at any age. This vibrancy could not be truer for Ernestine Shepherd, who started exercising at 56 when she desired more confidence as she aged. Now at 86, she is a personal trainer and professional bodybuilder with awe-inspiring strength and a youthful physique. She has even entered the Guinness Book of World Records as the world's oldest female bodybuilder. She enjoys doing motivational speaking while teaching her exercise classes. She says, "As long as I can move my arms, move my feet, and have presence of mind, I will continue this until my last breath is taken." Ernestine thrives on her routine. She notes that doing the same healthful things every day helps motivate consistency. Her dedication to her health as an active senior is inspiring. (Hill, 2021).

9

RELAXATION AND STRESS RELIEF IN THE COOL DOWN

> "Like all explorers, we are drawn to discover what's out there without knowing yet, if we have the courage to face it."
>
> — PEMA CHODRON (LIONS ROAR STAFF, 2017)

In the realm of Senior fitness, where flexibility, strength, and balance are prized qualities, a hidden gem is often overshadowed by the more dynamic aspects of exercise. This gem is the art of relaxation - a precious component that harmonizes the body, mind, and spirit. As we delve into the cool-down phase of Wall Pilates, we invite you to experience the gentle embrace of relaxation and stress relief, an essential element of your wellness journey.

Picture this: You have just completed a series of invigorating Wall Pilates exercises, feeling the strength and vitality surging through your body. Your muscles are awake, your posture refined, and your balance enhanced. Your heart rate is noticeably strong, and your breathing may be heavy. The effects of active movement can sometimes feel exhausting, yet they show us how we are powerful and capable. When we push ourselves to enjoy these challenging exercises, we learn to endure the challenges of keeping a healthy body. In this cool-down phase, we show gratitude for our bodies. Be proud of how far you've come!

This chapter is about creating your sanctuary, a tranquil oasis amongst the dynamic flow of your Wall Pilates routine. Here, we understand the significance of letting go, releasing the accumulated muscle tension, and unwinding the stress lingering from your life.

As we move from active movement to a restful calm, we create an awareness of our body. We are integrating all the healthful benefits of our practice into a highly mindful and relaxed state of being. As nonjudgemental observers, we scan the body to understand how these exercises affect us.

You will find a carefully crafted collection of techniques and exercises to promote physical relaxation and a sense of inner calm and rejuvenation. So please take a deep breath, let your worries disappear, and embark on a serene exploration of stress relief as we complete our practice.

BASIC RESTORATIVE COOL DOWN EXERCISES

We will begin our cool-down with a series of stretches that aim to promote gentle stretching, joint relief, and a slow decompression from the more challenging postures we do in our primary practice. These restorative poses help the body relax, and the muscles become supple to get the most out of your entire practice.

You have come so far in your practice; and these poses at the end are the feel good exercises. The stretches that remind us how nice exercises can feel in our body. We can end our workout day wanting to do it again tomorrow!

WRIST AND ARM STRETCH

Loosen the forearms, wrists, and hand muscles.

1. Hold your left arm straight out before you with your palm facing up.

2. With your right hand, hold the fingers of your left hand and pull them down and towards your body so that there is a stretch in the wrist and arms.

3. Hold to the count of 10.

4. Continue on the other side.

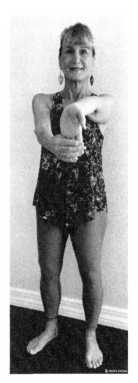

Step 2

CHEST STRETCH

Open the chest and shoulders.

1. Stand tall and take your arms behind your back, interlocking your fingers together.

2. Gently raise your arms upwards.

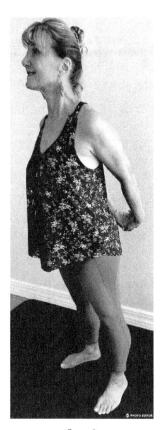

Step 2

3. Hold for the count of 10.

HIP TWIST

Movement in the hips for a full body stretch.

1. Stand tall with your arms relaxed at your sides.

- Ensure that you have enough clearance in a circle around your body so that you don't hit anything with your arms.

2. Begin the movement by rotating the body from side to side using your arms to facilitate the swinging movement and provide more twist in the hips and spine.

3. Continue to each side 10 times for a total count of 20 rotations.

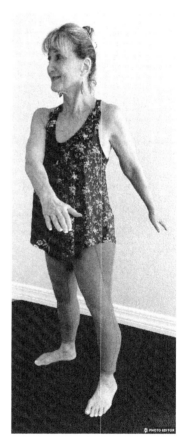

Step 2

HIP FLEXOR STRETCH

Opens the hips and stretches the front of the thighs.

1. Stand tall with your left hand on the wall in front of you.

2. Engage your abdominal muscles as you raise your left foot behind you.

3. Reach down and take hold of your foot with your left hand.

4. Using your hand, gently ease your foot and leg towards your body so that you feel a gentle stretch in the front of your thigh.

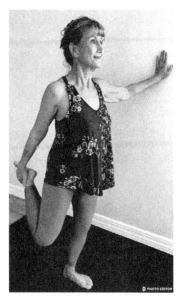

Step 4.

- Try not to arch your back.

5. Hold for the count of 10, breathing naturally.

6. Continue with the other leg.

7. Challenge Yourself:

- Hold your knees together and tilt the pelvis back for a deeper stretch.

HAMSTRING STRETCH

Stretching the back of the thighs.

1. Extend your left leg before you, ensuring both knees are parallel.

2. Keep your left leg straight and bend your right knee.

Place your hands on your right thigh for support as you bend over your leg.

- Be conscious of keeping your spine straight.

3. Feel the stretch in the back of your leg.

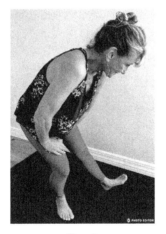

Step 3

4. Hold for the count of 10.

5. Continue on the other side.

ANKLE CIRCLES

Release tension in the ankle and calf.

1. Stand tall with your hand on the wall for support.

2. Raise your left foot off the ground.

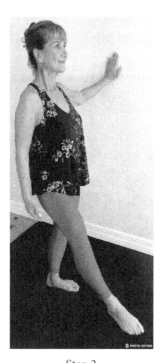

Step 2

3. Rotate it clockwise to the count of 5.

4. Rotate it counterclockwise to the count of 5.

5. Continue with the right foot.

TRICEPS STRETCH

Loosen the muscles in the arms and shoulders.

1. Cross the right arm over the chest and hold your upper arm with your left hand.

2. Pull your right arm gently towards your face while keeping the arm straight.

- Keep your hand relaxed and open.

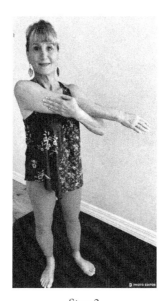

Step 2

3. You should feel a stretch in the upper arm and shoulder region.

4. Hold for a count of 10.

5. Continue with the left arm.

HIP OPENING STRETCH

Gentle release for the hips and upper legs.

1. Lay on the floor with your knees bent and the soles of your feet flat on the ground.

2. Lift your left foot and place the outside of your foot on your right knee.

3. Use your left hand to gently push your knee to feel a soft stretch in your hips and thigh.

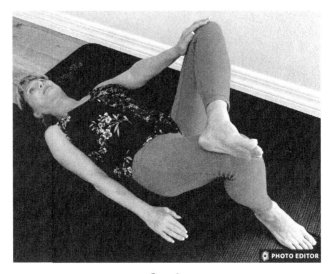

Step 3.

4. Hold for the count of 10.

5. Repeat with the other leg.

MINDFUL BREATHING

We always come back to breathe. Similar to how we started our journey, we will end our Pilates practice by focusing on our breath—the greatest constant in our day. When we return to the simple habit of mindful breathing, we can sink into a state of relaxation.

Pick one of these breathing techniques for the end of your practice and sit or lie down while you focus on the breath. These techniques are a great introduction to meditation. These practices help us be at peace with our thoughts, be more confident, reduce stress, and strengthen the mind-body connection. Here are 5 relaxing breathing techniques we can use during our cool-down.

DEEP BELLY BREATHING (DIAPHRAGMATIC BREATHING)

1. Sit or lie down in a comfortable position.

2. Place one hand on your chest and the other on your abdomen.

3. Inhale deeply through your nose, allowing your stomach to rise as you fill your lungs.

4. Exhale slowly through your mouth, letting go of tension.

5. Focus on the rise and fall of your abdomen.

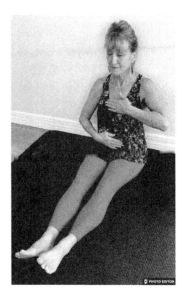

Step 2

6. Continue for several minutes, concentrating on each breath.

4-7-8 BREATHING (RELAXING BREATH)

Help calm the nervous system and reduce stress.

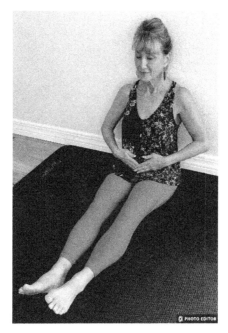

Step 1

1. Sit with your back straight and both hands on your abdomen.

2. Close your eyes and inhale quietly through your nose for a count of four.

3. Hold your breath for a count of seven.

4. Exhale entirely through your mouth, making a whooshing sound for a count of 8.

5. Repeat this cycle for 4-10 breaths.

BOX BREATHING (SQUARE BREATHING)

Helps regulate your breathing pattern and promotes relaxation.

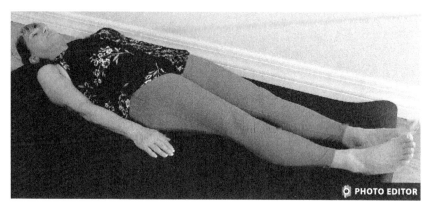

Step 1

1. Sit or lay down in a comfortable position.

2. Inhale through your nose for a count of four.

3. Hold your breath for a count of four.

4. Exhale through your mouth for a count of four.

5. Hold your breath for a count of four.

6. Repeat this cycle for 4-10 rounds, focusing on each step.

ALTERNATE NOSTRIL BREATHING (NADI SHODHANA)

Helps ease anxiety, lower blood pressure, and relax the mind.

1. Sit with your spine straight.

2. During this exercise, use your right thumb to close your right nostril and your right index finger to close your left nostril.

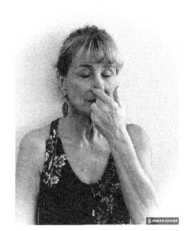

3. Inhale through your left nostril for a count of four.

4. Close your left nostril with your ring finger and release your right nostril.

Step 4

5. Exhale through your right nostril for a count of four.

6. Inhale through your right nostril.

7. Close your right nostril and release your left nostril.

8. Exhale through your left nostril.

9. Repeat this cycle for 4-10 breaths, focusing on the flow of breath.

VISUALIZATION TECHNIQUES

In the relaxing and refreshing experience of positive visualization techniques, come into balance with yourself. These following activities will elicit a mindful approach that is an excellent way to finish your Wall Pilates Exercises. Create a space for yourself that is free from distractions to set the stage for total relaxation.

Body Scan Visualization

1. Sit or lie down in a comfortable position.
2. Close your eyes and mentally scan your body, starting at your feet and working your way up your body to your head.
3. Notice any areas of tension, discomfort, or tightness.
4. As you identify these areas, visualize those muscles or joints relaxing and releasing tension.
5. Continue for 2-10 minutes.

Flowing River Visualization

1. In a comfortable sitting or lying down position, close your eyes.
2. Visualize your body as a flowing river.
3. As you Inhale, imagine that with each breath, the river's waters become calmer and smoother.
4. Exhale, visualizing any obstacles or tension in the river getting carried away by the gentle current.
5. Continue for 2-10 minutes.

Balloon Visualization

1. In a seated or lying position, close your eyes and imagine your body as a balloon.
2. Inhale deeply and visualize the balloon expanding with positive energy, filling you with lightness and a feeling of weightlessness.
3. Exhale slowly and imagine any worries, stress, or physical tension released into the atmosphere.
4. Continue for 2-10 minutes.

Mindful Gratitude Visualization

1. Reflect on your Wall Pilates session and your sense of overall well-being.
2. Visualize aspects of your health and your life that you are grateful for.
3. Express gratitude either silently or out loud for your strength, balance, and flexibility.

Relaxing Imagery Visualization

1. Find a comfortable position, lying down or sitting.
2. Close your eyes and visualize a serene environment like a meadow, garden, or cozy room.
3. Immerse yourselves in the imagery and experience. What are the sounds you hear? What colors do you see? What sensations contribute to a calming experience?

INSPIRING SENIOR BIO: PEMA CHODRON

The magic of mindfulness is continually coming back to the heart. Pema Chodron is an American Buddhist teacher interested in awakening compassion and kindness. Before becoming a Buddhist teacher, she led a relatively average life. It was not until a time of great suffering in her life when her ex-husband revealed he was having an affair, that Pema Chodron searched for a solution to cope with her pain.

Through the teachings of her mentor, she became supported by the Buddhist concepts of how suffering is inevitable, yet we can change how we respond to pain. These concepts empowered her to live in the present moment. She says, "Whatever life you're in is a vehicle for waking up." Through meditation and mindfulness practices, Pema Chodron has helped many people find peace in their suffering. "Meditation practice awakens our trust that the wisdom and compassion we need are already within us." (Lion's Roar Staff, 2017)

YOUR ONGOING WALL PILATES JOURNEY

"It's going to be a journey. It's not a sprint to get in shape."

— *KERRI WALSH JENNINGS (OLYMPIC WINNING VOLLEYBALL PLAYER.)*

Reflecting on where you started with Wall Pilates, look how far you've come! We hope you're feeling empowered and vibrant wherever you landed. You are not alone in your desire to improve your body and life. Countless others have benefited from these easy fitness exercises, and you can too!

Your path to wellness is not only paved with good intentions, but it's also lined with perseverance. We have the power to set the bar high for ourselves and overcome the challenges we face. Continuing your desire to better yourself and following through with manageable routines is a recipe for success with your fitness goals.

THE MAGIC OF MOTIVATION

To cultivate a mindset of continual improvement in our wellness habits, we need to find motivational factors that inspire us to participate.

Exercise is a gateway to our happiness endorphins. It helps us manage stress, elevates our mood, and gives us a natural boost in our desire to continue our Wall Pilates practice. This meditation in motion can alleviate any irritations from your day and help you focus on the incredible ability you still have to move and exercise a functioning body.

We can understand the subtle needs of our muscles when we slowly stretch and sculpt our Wall Pilates experience to be a personal journey for ourselves. Do what you love throughout your practice. Choose the postures that feel great and focus on how capable you are at them. Challenge yourself only when you are ready. Utilize our 21-day challenge to explore diverse postures that will advance your practice to the next level.

Stay open to new challenges; in doing so, you cultivate curiosity in the mind, allowing for renewed confidence and a feeling of vitality in spirit.

STAYING ACCOUNTABLE TO YOURSELF

We can set ourselves up for success with the right tools. Review the goals you set before you began your journey with Wall Pilates. Now that you have experience with some Wall Pilates poses, what realistic goals can you set for yourself?

How many days a week do you plan on working out?

How long will each work-out session be?

Make sure that your goals are manageable so that you can fulfill them. Over time, this will develop into a personalized Pilates routine that evolves with your skills.

Visualize your goals clearly to know what you are working towards during your Wall Pilates practice. Make your goals realistic and tangible. Goals could be losing 5 pounds, being able to move from point A to point B independently by yourself or being able to enhance your flexibility by being able to touch your toes. These goals help us hold ourselves accountable for actualizing visual results. Meeting set goals boosts your confidence level, and you can continue setting more challenging goals for yourself.

A JOURNEY TO INDEPENDENCE

This Wall Pilates journey can change the trajectory of your life far into the future. We can be active and engaged with the world as we become wiser through time. The changes that often occur as we age do not have to lead to dependence on outside help as we meet challenges in our abilities.

As we have learned from many of the spotlights on our inspiring elder bios, there is always time to step into our power. When we regain our mobility, it can transform how we look at ourselves. Our self-confidence becomes essential to being independent and able to take care of ourselves as time goes on. It may not be the reality for you right now, but with age comes more challenges to mobility. We must strengthen the body to be independent for as long as possible.

Now that you have committed to bettering your health through Wall Pilates, you will probably see the desire to enhance your wellness elsewhere, whether through nutrition, lifestyle choices, or emotional well-being. These positive choices can be incredibly beneficial for improved health and happiness.

We have experienced a well-rounded exercise routine together through this book. We started with the importance of safety and proper posture for everyday wellness. We then deepened our understanding of the body through deep breathing exercises and gentle warm-ups. We then challenged our bodies with exercises targeting our arms, backs, core, and legs. We always take the time to bring our bodies out of exercise mode by grounding our bodies in gentle cool-down stretches and using breathing and visualization to reduce anxiety and still the mind.

This Wall Pilates practice is the first stretch on a journey of independence in the golden age of your life. Thank you for embarking on this transformative experience with us, as we all ensure our lifelong well-being. Stay inspired by your goals! Find the motivation to integrate the practices in this book into your daily routine, and you will love the you that will emerge!

THE 21-DAY WALL PILATES CHALLENGE

Transform your well-being in **3** weeks!

Dive into a self-care routine by embarking on a transformative journey with Wall Pilates. You have made your way to understanding the importance Wall Pilates can have in your life. This challenge will incorporate all you have learned in this Wall Pilates book to put it into practice actively.

CHALLENGE OVERVIEW

Kickstart your daily practice by integrating just 10 Wall Pilates exercises into your daily routine. By setting your goals on short-term challenges, you can obtain the long-term results you desire. When you can commit yourself to this Wall Pilates Challenge, you will continue the practice after the challenge is over. Establishing a routine will help you become better acquainted with the Wall Pilates exercises by practicing them regularly, and your body will crave the delicious stretch and power you feel! It will become a seamless part of your daily life through the 10 minutes a day you commit to enhancing your health and wellness through Wall Pilates.

As we discussed in the first few chapters, create a dedicated space for your Wall Pilates so that you can easily practice each day. It is also essential to mentally ready yourself through positive affirmations and a determined mindset. Remember that you deserve to feel good about yourself. You have a body that you love to take care of.

Set goals for yourself that reflect your ability to commit and can ensure your success with the challenge. Create realistic expectations for yourself in completing your goals. Most importantly, do your best and have fun!

WEEK-BY-WEEK BREAKDOWN OF THE CHALLENGE

Week 1: Foundation and Familiarization

We will begin with an introduction to basic Wall-assisted Pilates exercises. We will focus on correct posture techniques, a supportive warm-up for joint flexibility, and gentle postures for increased mobility.

Week 2: Exploration and Confidence

We will integrate more diverse positions in the second week, focusing on our upper body and spinal strength. Use daily affirmations to build your beauty from the inside out!

Week 3: Intensification for Mastery

We will be working on exploring the boundaries of our abilities with postures increasing in intensity to feel the power our bodies can reach. We will focus on our core and lower body, incorporating some intermediate stretches, many of which require laying on a floor mat.

Week 1:
Building our Wall Pilates Foundation

Day 1 -Positive Posture

1. Even Balance
2. Wall Toe Touches
3. Pelvic Tilt
4. Neck Stretch
5. Neck Rotations
6. Spinal Rotations
7. Toe Lifts
8. Arm Reach
9. Hug a Tree
10. Ankle Circles
11. Diaphragmatic Breathing

Day 2 - Gentle Warm Up

1. Even Balance
2. Wall Toe Touches
3. Pelvic Tilt
4. Wall Heel Lift
5. Neck Rotations
6. Shoulder Rotations
7. Wrist Circles
8. Arm Lifts
9. Wall Calf Stretch
10. Forward Wall Lunges
11. Body Scan Visualization

Day 3 - Wake Up the Muscles

1. Even Balance
2. Wall Toe Touches
3. Sitting Stretch
4. Wall Arm Clock
5. Wrist Circles
6. Knee Lifts
7. Hug A Tree
8. Shoulder Stretch
9. Mini Squat
10. Hamstring Stretch
11. Deep Belly Breathing

Day 4 - Focus on the Feel-Good

1. Wall Toe Touches
2. Leg Balance
3. Spinal Rotations
4. Wrist Circles
5. Hip Opener Rotations
6. Toe Lifts
7. Forward Wall Lunge
8. Chest Stretch
9. Ankle Circles
10. Triceps Stretch
11. Flowing River Visualization

Day 5 - Balance and Alignment

1. Even Balance
2. Heel Lift
3. Wall Arm Clock
4. Neck Stretch
5. Neck Rotations
6. Knee Lifts
7. Toe Lifts
8. Arms Reach and Pull
9. Core Turn
10. Hamstring Stretch
11. 4-7-8 Breathing

Day 6 - Flexibility Flow

1. Wall Toe Touches
2. Sitting Stretch
3. Wall Heel Lift
4. Shoulder Rotations
5. Spinal Rotations
6. Wrist Circles
7. Hip Opener Rotations
8. Core turn
9. Chest Stretch
10. Triceps Stretch
11. Balloon Visualization

Day 7 - Vitality to Start Your Day

1. Reaching Stretch
2. Arm Lifts
3. Wall Cat-Cow
4. Shoulder Mobility
5. Pelvic Drop
6. Arm Circles
7. Arms Reach and Pull
8. Wall Side Bend
9. Wall Plank
10. Chest Stretch
11. Box Breathing

Great work on completing your first week of the Wall Pilates Challenge! You have experienced a gentle yet invigorating warm-up for your joints and muscles. This slow progression will prepare you for the increasingly challenging postures we will look at in Week 2, where we will focus on our arms and core. Congratulations on your motivation and dedication to yourself!

Week 2:
Gain Confidence Through Exploring Your Edge

Day 8- Life is Great!

1. Neck Stretch
2. Shoulder Rotations
3. Knee Lifts
4. Arm Circles
5. Shoulder Stretch
6. Arms Reach and Pull
7. Core Turn
8. Wall Plank
9. Chest Stretch
10. Triceps Stretch
11. Mindful Gratitude Visualization

Day 9 - My Body Feels Divine!

1. Spinal Rotations
2. Wrist Circles
3. Arm Lifts

4. Toe Lifts
5. Hug a Tree
6. Shoulder Mobility
7. Pelvic Drop
8. Wall Side Bend
9. Hip Flexor Stretch
10. Ankle Circles
11. Alternate Nostril Breathing

Day 10- I Am Capable of Anything I Put My Mind To.

1. Leg Balance
2. Neck Stretch
3. Wrist Circles
4. Hip Opener Rotations
5. Arms Reach and Pull
6. Wall Side Bend
7. Wall Plank
8. Spinal Stretch
9. Wrist and Arm Stretch
10. Chest Stretch
11. Relaxing Imagery Visualization

Day 11 - I am filled with Gratitude.

1. Knee Lifts
2. Toe Lifts
3. Arm Reach
4. Hug a Tree
5. Core Turn

6. Mountain Climber
7. Wall Forward Leg Lifts
8. Wall Side Leg Lifts
9. Chest Stretch
10. Hip Flexor Stretch
11. Deep Belly Breathing

Day 12 - Good Things Are Coming to Me.

1. Neck Rotations
2. Shoulder Rotations
3. Shoulder Mobility
4. Pelvic Drop
5. Spinal Stretch
6. Mini Squat
7. Wall Calf Stretch
8. Wrist and Arm Stretch
9. Hamstring Stretch
10. Ankle Circles
11. Body Scan Visualization

Day 13- I Believe in Myself.

1. Sitting Stretch
2. Reaching Stretch
3. Neck Stretch
4. Spinal Rotations
5. Arm Reach
6. Wall Push Up
7. Core Turn

8. Wall Plank with Leg Lift
9. Chest Stretch
10. Triceps Stretch
11. Flowing River Visualization

Day 14 - I Embrace My Power.

1. Arm Windows
2. Wall Cat-Cow
3. Pelvic Tilt
4. Arm Reach and Pull
5. Wall Push Up
6. Rowing the Boat
7. Wall Plank with Leg Lift
8. Spinal Stretch
9. Hip Flexor Stretch
10. Hamstring Stretch
11. 4-7-8 Breathing

The body has an incredible ability to adapt and persevere through even the most challenging of conditions. The mind power we put into a task can override all physical limitations we feel we may have. People can accomplish the most amazing transformations when they dedicate themselves to bettering their lives.

Great job sticking with the Wall Pilates Challenge! In the third week, we will explore many more spine-strengthening and lower-body toning exercises. This week includes more intermediate exercises to promote mastery of your body balance.

Feel free to repeat the affirmation mantras of the day while you exercise to enhance your mental well-being alongside your physical workout!

Week 3:
Stepping into Your Power Through Wall Pilates Mastery

Day 15- I Have Strength In Body and Mind

1. Wall Heel Lift
2. Spinal Rotations
3. Clock Exercise
4. Wall Plank with Leg Lift
5. Wall Bridge
6. Forward Wall Lunge
7. Wall Heel Squat
8. Wall Little Leg Lifts
9. Wall Roll Down
10. Ankle Circles
11. Balloon Visualization

Day 16- If I Work Hard, I'll Be Where I Want To Be.

- Rolling Posture
- Neck Stretch
- Wall Cat-Cow
- Pelvic Drop
- Wall Bridge
- Wall Crunches with Knee Pulls
- Wall Side Step

- Wall Back Leg Lifts
- Chest Stretch
- Hamstring Stretch
- Box Breathing

Day 17- I can do complex things.

1. Leg Balance
2. Arm Clock
3. Spinal Rotations
4. Wall Plank with Leg Lift
5. Wall Side Leg Lift
6. Wall Side-Step
7. Wall Sit
8. Hip Flexor Stretch
9. Mindful Gratitude Visualization

Day 18- I can make healthy choices.

1. Reaching Stretch
2. Shoulder Rotations
3. Wall Cat-Cow
4. Wall Push Ups
5. Mini Squat
6. Forward Wall Lunge
7. Wall Knee Bends
8. Wall Side Step
9. Wall Little Leg Lifts
10. Ankle Circles
11. Alternate Nostril Breathing

Day 19 – I love my body.

1. Neck Stretch
2. Hip Opener Rotations
3. Wall Cat-Cow
4. Mountain Climber
5. Table Top Wall Crunches
6. Wall Calf Stretch
7. Forward Wall Lunge
8. Wall Side Step
9. Wrist and Arm Stretch
10. Hamstring Stretch
11. Relaxing Imagery Visualization

Day 20 - I am worthy of health and happiness.

1. Arm Lifts
2. Knee Lifts
3. Wall Push Ups
4. Rowing the Boat
5. Core Turn
6. Wall Bridge
7. Wall Forward Lift
8. Wall Side Leg Lift
9. Wall Back Leg Lifts
10. Hip Twist
11. Deep Belly Breathing

Day 21 – Today and every day, I will do my best.

1. Reaching Stretch
2. Spinal Rotations
3. Wall Cat-Cow
4. Wall Push Up
5. Wall Crunches with Knee Pulls
6. Mini Squat
7. Wall Calf Stretch
8. Wall Heel Squat
9. Hip Opening Stretch
10. Ankle Circles
11. Body Scan Visualization

Thank you for your dedication to your health and for participating in kickstarting the transformation of your well-being. Now that you have structured your fitness experience in an attainable format, you can extend your practice beyond this challenge and into the future. Feel free to continue using these Wall Pilates routines to keep your practice active.

Share your success with others to inspire your friends and family to take charge of their health and well-being. Take your story to social media or involve another person in your workout to bring vibrancy into other's lives. You may be the catalyst for someone else's health transformation.

We are grateful to be able to inspire Seniors with a love for **Vibrancy as We Age**.

Keeping the Flame Alive

Now that you have unlocked the power of Wall Pilates, we would love to know about your Wall Pilates journey! Help us by sharing your newfound knowledge and guide other readers to the same transformative experience.

How You Can Keep the Flame Alive:

• *Leave Your Honest Opinion on Amazon: Your review isn't just words; it's a beacon for other readers, helping them find the information they want. Your passion for Wall Pilates can inspire others to embark on their own journey.*

• *Spread the Word: Share your thoughts on social media or recommend this book to friends and family. Your personal recommendation can spark curiosity and motivate someone to explore the benefits of Wall Pilates.*

• *Give the Gift of Knowledge: Consider gifting a copy to someone you care about. Your gesture might be the push they need to start a positive change in their life.*

Remember, the flame of knowledge doesn't flicker out when shared; it grows brighter. Thank you for being an integral part of this community and helping keep the flame alive.

Your contribution echoes far beyond these pages, and for that, we are sincerely grateful.

Until we meet again on the path of continued discovery,

Rachel and Leslie Haduch

REFERENCES

Pilates, J.H. (2012) *Return to Life Through Controlology*. Presentation Dynamics.

Pilates Foundation. (n.d.). The history of Pilates. Retrieved from https://www.pilatesfoundation.com/pilates/the-history-of-pilates/

Rhinebeck Pilates. (n.d.). Pilates history: Clara Pilates. Retrieved from https://www.rhinebeckpilates.com/pilates-history-clara-pilates/

Sixty and Me. (n.d.). Pilates strength training for women over 60. Retrieved from https://sixtyandme.com/pilates-strength-training/

Patti, Antonino PhD, Zangla Danielle. (2021, April 2). Physical Exercise and Prevention of Falls. *Medicine: Baltimore*, Volume 100 (13), https://www.ncbi.nlm.nih.gov/pmc/articles/PMC8021317/

Idavoy, Christie. (2021, September 3). How Pilates Helps to Prevent Falls. *Pilates Anytime*. https://www.pilatesanytime.com/blog/seniors/how-pilates-helps-prevent-falls

Menzies, Roxy. (2021, April 22). These 19 Benefits of Pilates Will Inspire You to Fire Up Your Core. *Healthline*. URLhttps://www.healthline.com/nutrition/pilates-benefits

Health Essentials. (2023, March 10) Pilates 101: What It Is and Health Benefits. *Cleveland Clinic*. https://health.clevelandclinic.org/everything-you-want-to-know-about-pilates/

Bedosky, Lauren. (2020, March 18) The At Home Pilates WorkOut for a Stronger Core. *Silver Sneakers*. https://www.silversneakers.com/blog/pilates-seniors-core-workout/

Gonul Babayigit Irez, Recep Ali Ozdemir . (2011, March) Integrating Pilates Exercise into an Exercise Program for 65+ year old women to prevent Falls. *Journal of Sports Science and Medicine*. Volume 10.1 https://www.researchgate.net/publication/258035528_Integrating_Pilates_Exercise_into_an_Exercise_Program_for_65_Year-Old_Women_to_Reduce_Falls

Health Library Articles. (2022, March 30) Diaphragmatic Breathing. *Cleveland Clinic*. https://my.clevelandclinic.org/health/articles/9445-diaphragmatic-breathing

Angell, Harry (2018, April 5) *Pilates for Living*. Bloomsbury Publishing.

Baxter, Sukie. (2019, April 16) 4 Tips to Improving Your Posture With

Embodied Mindfulness. *Chopra.* https://chopra.com/articles/4-tips-to-improving-your-posture-with-embodied-mindfulness

MedLine Plus. (n.d.) Guide To Good Posture. *National Library of Medicine.* https://medlineplus.gov/guidetogoodposture.html

Weisholtz, Drew. (2019, June 26) Meet the 85 Year Old Pole Vaulter Breaking Records. *Today.* Meet the 85-year-old pole vaulter breaking records (today.com)

Goldfarb, Kara. (2018, May 14.) He Was The Oldest Man to Climb Mt. Everest - 10 Years Later He Beat His Own Record. *All That's Interesting.* Yuichiro Miura Was The Oldest Man To Climb Mount Everest. Twice. (allthatsinteresting.com)

Blog, Yoga. (2016, September 9) Tao Porchon Lynch - Conversation with the Master. *Body In Balance Maui.* Tao Porchon-Lynch - Conversation with the Master - Body In Balance (bodybalancemaui.com)

Porchon-Lynch, Tao. (2015, October 2) *Dancing-Light: The Spiritual Side of Being Through The Eyes of a Modern Yoga Master.*

Averill, Graham. (2022, May 12) Pat Gallante-Charette Won't Stop Breaking Records. *Outside.* Pat Gallant-Charette Won't Stop Breaking Records (outsideonline.com)

Blogify Spot. (2023, June 4) 10 Powerful Core Pilates Exercises to Help ReIgnite Your Abdominal Strength. https://blogifyspot.com/10-powerful-wall-pilates-core-exercises/#Exercise_1_Wall_Roll-Up

Long, Robin. (2014, November 7) Pilates for Beginners : Part 4 Spinal Rotations. *LindyWell.* https://lindywell.com/pilates-beginners-part-four-spinal-rotation/

Pilates On Demand With Lindsay. (2023) Get Toned Abs With This Beginner Wall Pilates Plank WorkOut. *YouTube.* https://www.youtube.com/watch?v=-ykX98DcUi8

Paden, Linda. (2014, December 2) Idiots Guide To Pilates. *DK Publishing.*

Mukhwana, Jeremy. (2023, November) Wall Pilates Exercises for Beginners, Seniors and Anyone Looking for a Change. *Better Me.* https://betterme.world/articles/wall-pilates-exercises

Hannah Rae Training. (2021) Five Minute Shoulder Opening: Pilates On the Wall. *YouTube.* https://www.youtube.com/watch?v=sJfX2cbjNNw

Yes2Next. (2023) 5 Wall Exercises For Seniors and Beginners. *YouTube.* https://www.youtube.com/watch?v=HHnpgHNkLcE

Bedosky, Lauren. (2020, March 18) The At-Home Pilates Workout For a

Stronger Core. *Silver Sneakers.* https://www.silversneakers.com/blog/pilates-seniors-core-workout/

Butler, S.L. (2017, October 16) Harriet Thompson, Oldest Woman to Finish a Marathon, Dies at 94. *Runner's World.* https://www.runnersworld.com/news/a20862554/harriette-thompson-oldest-woman-to-finish-a-marathon-dies-at-94/

Kumar, Aishwarya. (2017, June 6) Meet the 94 Year Old Woman Who Can Hang With You In a Half-Marathon. *ESPN.* https://www.espn.com/sports/endurance/story/_/id/19562514/half-marathon-harriette-thompson-becomes-oldest-woman-complete-half-marathon

Fisher, M.Z. (2022, July 6) At 92 Years Young, the Iron Nun is Still Running. *TriAthlete.* https://www.triathlete.com/culture/people/at-91-years-young-the-iron-nun-is-still-running/

Crouch, Michelle. (2019, October 16) Inspiring Stories From Later-In-Life Athletes. *AARP.* https://www.aarp.org/health/healthy-living/info-2019/inspiring-older-athletes.html

Wamaitha, Lilian. (2021, April 26) 50 Inspiring Senior Fitness Quotes To Get You Moving. *Loaids.* https://loaids.com/senior-fitness-quotes/

Hill, Jordan. (2021, June 15) Ernestine Shepard at 85: A Day In the Life of World's Oldest Female Body Builder. *Black Doctor. Org.* https://blackdoctor.org/ernestine-shepherd-day-in-the-life-video/

Lion's Roar Staff. (2017, July 14) The Best of Pema Chodron: Life, Quotes and Books. *Lions Roar.* https://www.lionsroar.com/pema-chodron/#quotes

Lion's Roar Staff. (2016, March 14) A Beginner's Guide to the Teachings of Pema Chodron. *Lion's Roar.* https://www.lionsroar.com/a-beginners-guide-to-the-teachings-of-pema-chodron/

Dienstman, A. M. (2019, January 21) How to Cope With Suffering According to the Buddha. *Goodnet.* https://www.goodnet.org/articles/how-to-cope-suffering-according-buddha

Mayo Clinic Staff. (2022, August 3) Exercise and Stress: Get Moving to Manage Stress. *Mayo Clinic.* https://www.mayoclinic.org/healthy-lifestyle/stress-management/in-depth/exercise-and-stress/

Cronkleton, Emily. (2023, May 24) What are the benefits and risks of Alternate Nostril Breathing? *Healthline. Alternate Nostril Breathing: Benefits, How To, and More* (healthline.com)